LIVING WITH THE LONG-TERM EFFECTS OF CANCER

Acknowledging Trauma and other Emotional Challenges

Dr Cordelia Galgut

Illustrated by Louise Bourgeois

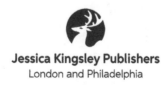

Jessica Kingsley Publishers
London and Philadelphia

Where requested, the names and biographical details of people featured in this book have been changed to make them anonymous.

The information contained in this book is not intended to replace the services of trained medical professionals or to be a substitute for medical advice. You are advised to consult a doctor on any matters relating to your health, and in particular on any matters that may require diagnosis or medical attention.

First published in 2020
by Jessica Kingsley Publishers
73 Collier Street
London N1 9BE, UK
and
400 Market Street, Suite 400
Philadelphia, PA 19106, USA

www.jkp.com

Library of Congress Cataloging in Publication Data
A CIP catalog record for this book is available from the Library of Congress

British Library Cataloguing in Publication Data
A CIP catalogue record for this book is available from the British Library

ISBN 978 1 78592 462 0
eISBN 978 1 78450 839 5

Printed and bound in Great Britain

CONTENTS

ACKNOWLEDGEMENTS

My thanks to:

- Elen Griffiths and Maddy Budd at Jessica Kingsley Publishers
- Simon Crompton
- Mitzi Blennerhassett
- Professor Diana Greenfield
- Louise Bourgeois
- Deirdre King
- Those who agreed to be interviewed for this book.

Also, my thanks to:

- Dr John Conibear
- Jane Fior
- Michael Galgut
- Dr Peter Galgut
- Dr Frances Goodhart
- Mr Dimitri Hadjiminas
- Louise Johnson
- Professor Vik Khullar
- Liz Lane
- Dr Richard Marley
- Ruth McCurry
- Ben Parker
- Wendy Rangeley
- Jonathan Rée

- Anne Vadgama
- All those I have talked to in passing, whose words have informed my thinking and thereby the content of this book
- And last, but not least, to Kate, for doing all that she could to support me with this project, and for all her help and support over the last 38 years.

INTRODUCTION

This book is for a wide audience. Moreover, given that estimates predict that one in two of us will receive a diagnosis of cancer in our life times (Cancer Research UK 2015), or will be affected by it second hand, in a sense this book is for us all, especially since these days growing numbers live on after a cancer diagnosis (Macmillan Cancer Support 2019).

In the first instance, however, this book is for the many living with and beyond cancer, coping with its long-term effects,[1] both physical and emotional, whether they be more or less severe. I hope this book offers new and welcome support and insights for those of you in these situations, by delving into areas that are not often spoken about but that affect many of us.

In revealing some of the actual reality of what we endure, I hope that you will feel that your suffering is understood and taken seriously. I also hope that reading my stories, and those of others who have long-term effects, whose quotes I

---

[1] For the purposes of this book, 'long-term effects' are defined as any symptoms that started after diagnosis and treatment and that don't go away, whether they are static or have got worse, be they physical or emotional. Additionally, the effects of cancer that were not present after the initial diagnosis and treatments, that come on either slowly or more suddenly, including a secondary diagnosis, are included.

have used throughout the book, will confirm that you are not alone.[2] I trust that you will also take heart from the fact that I am publicising these issues. In addition, I am hopeful that the practical support in this book will help, although I cannot claim that this is a self-help book to any significant degree.[3]

This book is also for the families and friends of those living with the long-term effects of cancer, and also for anyone interested in this subject. I hope that the book informs and supports this group of people too.

Last, but not least, this book is for those who work in cancer care at every level and in every area. I know that there are many committed people working in this field who make a huge difference to the quality of life of people coping with cancer's long-term effects, in spite of limited resources. I really hope that this book raises awareness of and validates the work that you do.

I trust that this book will also serve to enlighten those in the cancer field and related ones who are keen to know more about the psychological and physical long-term effects of cancer, and

---

2   I, interviewed, talked to, emailed etc., a fair number of people, either formally or informally, for the purposes of this book – approximately a hundred. My rationale for doing so was to gauge, from their words, what the issues are that have preoccupied them in relation to the long-term effects of cancer. I interviewed both those who suffer from cancer's long-term effects, across a variety of cancers, and, additionally, professionals working with those affected. I also talked to a few people who were both long-term sufferers and healthcare professionals, and to some working in related areas; for example, people working for charities. Almost everyone wanted to remain anonymous when quoted in this book, which was confirmation of what I already suspected. At this time in the UK the subject of this book remains a contentious, highly charged area. People wanted their views aired, but for the most part were not willing to risk using their real names or be too explicit about where they worked, etc., a stance I fully understand, given the context.

3   *The Cancer Survivor's Companion* (2011), written by fellow psychologist, Dr Frances Goodhart, and health journalist, Lucy Atkins, is a good accompaniment to this book, in that its focus is on offering practical support for coping with feelings that arise after cancer. Additionally, my handbook, *Emotional Support Through Breast Cancer* (Galgut 2013a), offers specific practical support for those with breast cancer.

that it will contribute to a body of knowledge about the reality of life years after diagnosis and treatment/s.

I am also hopeful that it will encourage debate, by highlighting little known issues that need serious and prompt consideration, in order to improve the quality of life for those who suffer long term. Their needs are currently not being adequately met in the UK and very possibly elsewhere in the world too.

A dual perspective

I chose to write this book from the dual perspective I have, as a psychologist who had breast cancer and who is coping with the long-term effects of treatments I received 15 years ago. While this seems more honest to me, I imagine that there will be those who criticise me for it. I am hopeful that those who read this book, including healthcare professionals will recognise that in embracing my 'insider' bias, I am potentially adding breadth and depth to what I write, rather than the reverse, not least because, as Liz, who has had cancer, says, 'The professional voice is usually heard above all others.' In writing from my dual perspective, I am hoping to right that balance a little, as well as support others living long-term with cancer's effects, who feel validated when health professionals and others speak out from their dual perspectives.

I also hope to contribute to the debate about whether it is possible to be both ill and vulnerable, and powerful and productive, both in the work domain and elsewhere. Obviously, I believe it is possible to inhabit and embody both states, and trust that I am living proof of that, although I am aware that others might disagree.

Limitations

There will, of course, be distinct limits to the ground I can cover in this book and there will subsequently be a fair number of omissions, for which I apologise in advance. This is also a relatively short book, which further limits the details I can include. Frustratingly, I have only been able to scrape the surface of some issues, each of which warrants a book itself.

Furthermore, while I am assuming some commonality of experience between cancers longer term I also acknowledge that there will be many differences too for example, a man's experience of prostate cancer is not likely to be the same as a woman's experience of breast cancer. Equally, people's long-term experience of the same cancer will very possibly differ as well as chime with others' experiences. I also acknowledge that my personal experience of cancer is limited to breast cancer.

Additionally, since I am a psychologist and not a medical person, this book's primary focus is on the psychological impact of cancer in the long term and not the physical, although clearly the two are inseparably intertwined – each one affects the other, and many physical effects are mentioned in this book.

There are also differing opinions about what a book about the long-term effects of cancer should cover. For example, out of respect to those with a secondary diagnosis, where there is spread to bones and organs, some would say that I should not even attempt to consider this area since I do not have a secondary diagnosis myself. They might well say that this aspect should be covered separately in a book dedicated solely to secondary cancer sufferers' issues and needs. Others might say that my lack of first-hand experience of secondary cancer is not such a problem. They might say that on the continuum of cancer, with diagnosis at one end and the possibility of death at the other, since most cancers can spread elsewhere in the body at any point, a secondary diagnosis can be a long-term effect, albeit a very severe and devastating one.

This is obviously a complex area, and I am not exactly sure where I sit regarding it. However, in my personal opinion, whether our diagnosis is primary or secondary, one thing many of us do suffer from, to a greater or lesser degree, is lack of awareness of our situation and lack of help and support with it. So it could be argued that, to this extent, primary and secondary cancer 'survivors'[4] are all in the same boat, and I have tried to reflect this in what follows, as well as I am able.

Additionally, I apologise if I appear to make unfair judgements about any person or group of people. And I apologise if I seem to imply at any point in this book that I think cancer is the only life-threatening illness that has long-term effects.[5] If I appear to do so for either the former or the latter, please understand that this is not my intention, which is rather to highlight and unpick, as best as I can, the complex issues related to the long-term effects of cancer, for the benefit of everyone concerned – no more and no less.

---

4   See also footnote 1. The word 'survivor', when used to describe someone who has lived beyond cancer diagnosis and treatment, is controversial, and I have tried not to over-use it in this book, except in an ironic way. It tends to be associated with 'brave' people 'battling' cancer, and other ways of describing living with and beyond cancer that, for many of us, do not describe the reality of our experiences either adequately or accurately.

5   I am taking it as read that many people with cancer have other conditions too, that pre-existed their cancer diagnosis, either life-threatening or not, as well as those they have developed as a result of cancer. However, I do not make the assumption in this book that a pre-existing condition always makes long-term effects more likely. An assumption I do make, however, is that coping with one condition is likely to make coping with the other/s harder.

CHAPTER 1

WHY IS THIS BOOK NEEDED?

Nobody seems to accept that I'm struggling like this so long after my cancer treatment. I need help, but nobody understands. They expect me to be back to normal, but how can I be? (Suky, diagnosed with bowel cancer five years ago)

'You should be grateful to be alive'

The mismatch

Despite growing and compelling evidence to the contrary, some of which has been available to the public for several years now; for example, Macmillan Cancer Support's report, *Cured – But at What Cost?* (2013a), there seems to be little acceptance in the world at large, including within healthcare, that large numbers of those of us who live beyond either a primary or secondary diagnosis routinely suffer a variety of nasty, long-term side effects, both emotional and physical.

Contrary to received wisdom on the subject, these side effects can also worsen over time, not get better. In addition to suffering in ways that quite often seriously affect people's quality of life, anyone living beyond, or with, cancer, also has to endure a huge mismatch between their lived reality of life after diagnosis/es and treatment/s and how others, and indeed they themselves, have been told life would be.

Furthermore, the 'you're lucky you're alive' school of thought that those who live on are often enough bombarded by – although understandable; for example, in the face of people losing loved ones to cancer – is an immense source of extra stress for anyone struggling after cancer diagnosis and treatment. Such judgements ring in our ears as we limp through, emotionally and physically, often suffering in silence lest we are also told we are, for example, 'exaggerating' or 'responding abnormally'.

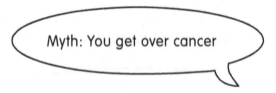

Myth: You get over cancer

As someone diagnosed with breast cancer twice in 2004, aged 48/49, I was told repeatedly that I should expect to be back to normal a year or so after my surgeries and initial treatments. It was, therefore, an enormous shock to me that I didn't return to normal, either psychologically or physically. Indeed, the four years of adjuvant chemotherapy I had (after the three months of daily radiotherapy), starting a few months after my initial treatment, were totally miserable ones.

'Am I losing it?'

I remember thinking, 'Am I going mad because I'm being told that the way I feel is not normal?' I even remember being told I was over-reacting by a doctor to whom I was explaining that I was frightened of recurrence! In the midst of this, I was also told by another doctor that they would much rather have cancer than chronic fatigue syndrome (CFS). This was based on a belief that you recover from cancer and get back to your normal, active self, whereas with CFS – which as I know from personal experience is an awful condition – you do not. While I wouldn't question this doctor's assumption about CFS, I did and still would maintain that for many of us, cancer is not a diagnosis we can ever 'get over'.

There are many reasons for this, which I will touch on in this chapter and expand on in later chapters, using others' words as well as my own. Broadly speaking, my assertion is that it is fairly impossible to 'get over' cancer when, for most of us, we know it can return at any point. Furthermore, contrary to what many would expect, it is a rare person who has had a cancer diagnosis who doesn't endure longer-term effects of some sort, both physical and emotional (Crompton 2018; Macmillan Cancer Support 2017). And as I mentioned earlier, these physical and emotional effects are, inevitably, inseparably intertwined.

I was particularly struck by this doctor's assuredness that they were right, comparing CFS and cancer in the way they did. I remember saying to them that I wasn't so sure that there was as much of a difference as they were asserting. This was because there was more than a dawning awareness in me that some of the effects from, for example, radiotherapy and surgery, and maybe even the cancer itself, that I had been told would get better over time, were, in fact, doing the reverse.

I wasn't alone, after all

When I started to write about my observations that things were getting worse for me, both emotionally and physically, and started to have this writing published, I was relieved to find that I was not alone experiencing what I was in relation to the longer-term effects. I particularly remember writing a piece for *Breast Cancer Care News* in 2007 (Galgut 2007a) about four years after the end of my last radiotherapy, and being somewhat unsure how either those who had had a diagnosis of breast cancer or my healthcare profession colleagues would respond. This was because I risked going out on a limb, saying that, contrary to what my training in psychology had taught me, in relation to life post trauma, I wasn't responding as I was supposed to. Instead, I was still living on a knife's edge, terrified of recurrence, even though I had early stage breast cancer and my prognosis was very good.

'It's only you who feels like this'

I was also trepidatious because no medical person or anyone else involved in cancer care was saying anything other than that I should expect the reverse of what I was actually experiencing. Indeed, I was being told by them that my ongoing anxiety was excessive and that my reactions, both emotional and physical, were unusual. I just assumed that I must be a rare case, on some level, not helped by my training in psychology and counselling, which had tended to support the 'you should be over major trauma in a year' school of thought.

However, the response to my piece in *Breast Cancer Care News* was overwhelming, with many women writing to me to tell me how relieved they were that a psychologist, who also knew what breast cancer was like first hand, was echoing how they felt, and what a relief it was that they were 'normal'. So they, like me, had been feeling that they were the only ones feeling as they did. Very movingly, a few women told me that hearing that it was normal to feel as they did had even alleviated their suicidal feelings.

Quite a number of women also urged me to keep speaking out on their behalf, because, much as they wanted to, they didn't dare to for fear of being labelled 'mad' and/or 'abnormal'. They also worried that speaking out would compromise their care, as it might affect how their doctors and nurses behaved towards them if they found out what they really thought.

This was a turning point for me, as I started to assimilate, on a deeper level, how this tendency of the medical profession and other healthcare colleagues to label anxious patients 'abnormal' when they are just exhibiting normal human, emotional responses can be unhelpful psychologically. What I mean by this is health professionals and others saying, 'It's only you' rather than 'I know you're not alone, experiencing what you are.'

People with other cancers often feel likewise

Since then, I have spoken to many others putting up with longer-term effects across a number of different cancers. I have found much common ground, even though treatments for different cancers vary. The views that those affected hold are often similar, confirming this mismatch between how we are supposed to feel after cancer and how life actually is.

And the effects of this mismatch on those suffering the long-term effects of cancer can be emotionally devastating, sometimes even more so than the physical effects they endure. Therefore, *this mismatch must be challenged* now more than ever before, as more and more people live years beyond diagnosis, with or without recurrence.

Why this mismatch exists also needs investigating, and *what can be done about it* explored – hence the need for this book.

Truth: The effects of cancer endure

When I started to have the courage of my convictions and began to speak out more, within healthcare circles I found that healthcare professional colleagues could be defensive.

They also tended to get impatient with me when I spoke from my dual perspective, as both a psychologist and as a woman who had been diagnosed with two breast cancers. On one occasion, after I had given a talk from this dual perspective, I was confronted by a colleague who told me that I couldn't be both psychologist and patient at the same time; that I should speak as either one or the other. When I asked why not, I was told that when I spoke from my patient perspective, I was lessening the impact of my argument, because I couldn't be objective. My reaction was to say that I didn't think we could ever be objective, from any perspective, but that comment fell on deaf ears.

I was also told that people felt criticised when I spoke from my patient perspective. I tried to explain that I was not criticising anyone but that having supported women with breast cancer prior to having it myself and thinking I was doing a good enough job, I was shocked to find that I had made some seriously inaccurate assumptions. No doubt the people I was supporting had indeed realised but were too polite to tell me. I said I felt it was my duty to speak out about what I had learned from being in the patient's shoes, and hoped people would be interested in my new insights. Unfortunately, the response I got was that I was over-reacting.

Sadly, this kind of attitude remains quite prevalent within healthcare, and it is one that needs constant challenging in order to improve patient care across the board. I do understand this stance in that it is, in part at least, a form of self-protection. I think it is also more insidious in origin, as it is part of a medical model, paternalistic attitude to patients, that most of the people I know in healthcare would now consider outmoded, unsavoury and entirely unnecessary.

Certainty breeds inaccuracy

'You're over-anxious. It's not normal. You should be over cancer by now and getting on with your life'

Received wisdom about how life should be after a cancer diagnosis can be a real force to contend with. As an example of this, I remember clearly that when my first book, which I had written from my dual perspective, *The Psychological Impact of Breast Cancer*, came out in 2010 (Galgut 2010), six years after my first diagnosis, a critic suggested that I was abnormal for still suffering, both emotionally and physically, so long after diagnosis, despite the fact that there were many examples in the book of others who felt as I did. The critic was someone who had not had breast cancer herself, as far as I was aware, although she was professing to be an authority on the psychological effects of breast cancer. I remember being very struck and somewhat shocked by how clear she was that her views were the right ones and that mine were ridiculous, and also by her entrenched, closed stance.

A force to contend with

This critic's extremely negative judgement was a baptism of fire for me and a good lesson in what I was up against, challenging the cancer establishment in the way I was. I knew the critic was not alone in her views about how life should be after cancer, and, in a way, I understood her stance. Before having breast cancer myself I had been closer to her opinion, both in terms of how I viewed mental health post trauma and also how I viewed life after breast cancer. This person had very likely felt criticised by my changed stance, and I understood well enough why – I was questioning received wisdom about how life is during and after cancer in a way that was challenging her long-held beliefs.

A high mountain to climb

Sadly, I have encountered a fair number of other negative reactions, both within and outside the healthcare world, in the process of highlighting the mismatch between what conventional wisdom says about what life is like after cancer and its actual reality for many of us.

I particularly remember trying to work with an organisation when writing my second book, *Emotional Support Through Breast Cancer* (2013a). I wrote this book because a number of women with a breast cancer diagnosis had urged me to do so, as they were so fed up with people telling them they should be 'over' breast cancer after a year or so and that they should have 'moved on'. To say it was a frustrating experience working with this particular organisation was an understatement.

This frustration arose from a disagreement between us about how much emotional upset those affected experience after breast cancer diagnosis and treatment. They tended to think that it was a minority of women who had longer-term problems, both psychological and physical, and my publishers and I believed the contrary. In the end, we decided that we couldn't collaborate with the organisation because our views and those of the organisation differed so much that it would be impossible to achieve a good outcome.

Interestingly, when my handbook was published, reviews confirmed large numbers suffering longer term after breast cancer, both emotionally and physically. For example, Macmillan Cancer Support asked 24 people who had breast cancer to do a detailed review of the book – 13 gave it the top rating of 5 stars and 8 gave it 4 stars, agreeing that suffering continues after diagnosis and treatment. A boost to my ego aside, it was a great relief to get some confirmation that what word of mouth and my own experience had led me to believe had been confirmed in this way.[1]

The book also received an award from the British Medical Association in 2014, which was very gratifying, not least because it showed that there are those in the medical world whose attitudes are not so entrenched, and that there are listening ears within medicine.

It's still a high mountain, though

Nevertheless, as I write this book, the mountain is still very much there, its face as steep and treacherous as ever, due, in part, to the influence that a certain entrenched faction still has in the cancer world. As Kari, a nurse working in the cancer field, told me recently,

> I wouldn't dare challenge these people who have been around for years as they're much older and more powerful than me and I might lose my job, but I see them with patients and I cringe sometimes. They think they know best and in some ways they do, but they miss so much because they're so closed-minded and patients suffer because of it. It's hard to watch sometimes.

Perhaps it is now time to push the boundaries of what we are prepared to talk about and confront in relation to the long-term effects of cancer. This is the purpose of my book – a timely contribution to the debate, I hope, and to an increasing body of knowledge available on this issue.

Summary

For those suffering the long-term effects of cancer, it can help if:

---

1   See www.emotionalsupportthroughbreastcancer.co.uk/bookreviews.html

- We can remind ourselves that there is often a clear mismatch between what we are told about how life after diagnosis will be, longer term, and how it actually is for many of us.
- We can allow ourselves to validate our own experience of cancer's long-term effects and remind ourselves that we are definitely not alone in feeling as we do, and we don't have to feel guilty that we have survived.
- We can have the confidence to challenge those who are not in our position about the reality of living long term with cancer's effects, this can improve life to some degree, psychologically at least.

Speaking out can be empowering – though there is no imperative to do so, if you don't feel like it. Saying some version of the following to someone who belittles what you are coping with might help, though these are just suggestions. I imagine that there are many more that you can think of:

- They cannot really know how it feels if they are not in your situation. You know you are not alone in experiencing what you do.
- You would appreciate them suspending their judgement and listening to your lived experience.
- You are alive, but the quality of your life has diminished (a lot), and this is hard to cope with.

For healthcare professionals, family, friends, etc., it can be really helpful if you tell your patient/partner/friend, etc. that you:

- understand that life is varying degrees of hard for them
- want to know what they are going through
- accept that there is a mismatch between how healthcare or society views life after a diagnosis of cancer and how many actually experience it

- know that life after cancer diagnosis/es is often harder than we are led to believe it is
- take your hat off to them for coping as they do
- won't always get it right, but you want to try
- want your patient/partner/friend to tell you if you don't get it right.

Obviously, a partner or friend might want to go further than a healthcare professional can, realistically, to take on all of the above. However, these suggestions remain applicable whether you are working with a patient or supporting someone coping longer term, as their partner, family member, friend, etc.

CHAPTER 2

WHY DO WE STRUGGLE TO ACCEPT THAT LONG-TERM EFFECTS EXIST?

I have asked myself this question many times. Why does society at large, and why do even healthcare professionals, mostly insist on a version of life after diagnosis that is essentially inaccurate, since it plays down the reality of these effects? This is a complex question that runs very deep, and the reasons below are by no means exhaustive.

Reason 1: Entrenched attitudes

'I've been doing this job for years. I know better'

Entrenched attitudes and closed minds are as endemic in healthcare as they are in the world at large. I can certainly sympathise with those in healthcare who get angry and defensive with those who challenge their entrenched thinking; it's very uncomfortable. However, the maintenance of an ethos that promotes the superiority of entrenched thinking and conventional wisdom over different and new perspectives and understandings can cause significant emotional disruption to people. How, you may ask?

Macmillan's *Am I Meant to Be Okay Now?* (Macmillan Cancer Support 2017) cites many examples, from a medical context and elsewhere, of people who have been affected by these kinds of attitudes. For example, Florencia, who finished treatment for bone cancer 21 months ago, says, 'They [medical people] think that once you've finished treatment, you're okay.' Furthermore, Chris, from the same Macmillan report, says, 'Having finished treatment for head and neck cancer, 10 months ago, people say to me, "I bet you wake up every morning feeling glad to be alive." You know, it can't be further from the truth.'

Unfortunately, the net result is too often, although understandable, that those affected by cancer feel they've failed because, as Frances, quoted in the same report, who finished treatment for Hodgkin lymphoma four years ago, says, 'You feel like you're a failure and you've failed to bounce back in the way you think you should.'

'Cancer patients are not rational'

Although not all healthcare professionals approach cancer patients or patients in general in this way, there is a tendency to do so. The medical model of healthcare that is still prevalent in the UK tends to infantilise and/or diminish patients' views. They are ill and therefore not able to step back from their own situation and assess it accurately. Therefore, any patient complaining of long-term effects can easily be dismissed as irrational, over-reacting or delusional.

As Melanie, diagnosed with bowel cancer six years ago, said,

I can't believe how the doctor treated me when I tried to tell him about the problems I've had since the surgery and the treatments. He just dismissed what I was saying and said it was nothing to do with any cancer treatment and that I was overwrought and needed a rest and that that would help, but I know other people who have the pain I have and the incontinence and he treated me like I was six years old with no right to an opinion. It really annoyed me. I wasn't upset before I saw him but I was afterwards. And I need some help but I have no idea where to get it.

'I listened, but I didn't hear. I looked, but I didn't see'

As the healthcare professional I had been for years, I admit that I, too, was guilty of closing my ears and eyes to things that challenged me too much. Rather, I listened, but I didn't hear. I looked, but I didn't see. It wasn't until I had breast cancer myself, twice, that I realised how ignorant I had been about the reality of breast cancer diagnosis and treatments. Before that, in truth, I was too stuck in a rut to find out more. And I understand why others are too. However, I think we have both a professional and ethical duty to face our own entrenched attitudes, in this case about the long-term effects of cancer (or admit it if we can't), or we are not likely to be of much use to anyone coping with cancer's effects.

'I was too frightened'

I was also too frightened of breast cancer and the possibility that I might get it myself to listen properly to those I was supporting emotionally. I told myself I was listening and did understand well enough, but my fear got in the way. Then I got the disease I was so terrified of getting and was catapulted into new and alien territory. Life changed. I changed. It's not that I am less frightened of cancer now – having cancer hasn't cured me of that – but I have had to face it head on and it is familiar territory now, 15 years later.

I now understand that which I could not have understood prior to getting it. Nonetheless, I could have risked trying to understand better. I could have confronted my own fear more than I did, and I could have admitted to myself and to those I was supporting emotionally that, first, I didn't know what they were going through but that I wanted to listen and understand as well as I could, and second, that breast cancer scared me. From my current vantage point, I know that these disclosures can often be well received by those engaging in therapy and are well worth risking.

Reason 2: General fear of cancer

'Nobody really wants to think about cancer, let alone its long-term effects'

People are constantly being told that half of us alive today will get a diagnosis of cancer (Cancer Research UK 2015). This is a scary prediction and it would take an unusual person, probably a robot, not to be very frightened by it, those working in healthcare included. Furthermore, the history of cancer that has been passed down through the generations, that cancer kills, remains in our collective psyche. Most of us know people who have died of cancer. Those who have already had one or more diagnosis/es live in fear of another, and of death. And, of course, the language/phrases we use in English do nothing to dispel our fears; for example, 'It's like a cancer in our society.' Without meaning to, using phrases such as this can risk reinforcing our fear and terror of a cancer that always spreads and always kills its host.

Of course, these days cancer doesn't always kill. On the contrary, it is being talked about more and more as a chronic condition, hence the need for this book! But then many of us know people who have had a very hard time enduring treatments for cancer. And I am often told that people who haven't had cancer fear the treatments more than anything else, even though sometimes they can be less harsh than previously.

Reason 3: Attitudes of 'survivors'

'I shouldn't be feeling this way'

Those of us who have had a diagnosis, or multiple diagnoses, of cancer are generally no less susceptible to a, 'I shouldn't complain' version of life after treatment than healthcare professionals (Macmillan Cancer Support 2017). Cancer patients are no different in relation to the attitudes that most of us have been conditioned to believe are the right way to think and act. This is, namely, to play down our thoughts and emotions, especially if they are negative. We can therefore give others the impression we are enduring less than we are.

It takes a brave person to go against the grain and say they are struggling, that survival isn't all roses and, on the contrary, that life is bleak. I know myself how much wrath someone who risks speaking out can be on the receiving end of. People frequently think we should just be grateful. It is often much easier to keep quiet, especially given how conflicted many of us will feel about speaking out, since we will probably be fighting our conditioned responses telling us to 'keep quiet' and to 'think ourselves lucky'.

There is also survivor guilt. I can't count how many times, over the last 15 years, I have been told by people from all walks of life, including my own colleagues, that I'm fortunate that I've survived and then seen someone's eyes glaze over when I've talked about how hard my life is coping with the long-term effects of cancer. Even though I know I'm telling the truth, it can be extremely hard for me to validate my own feelings, although people expect me to be able to, because of my profession. I can find myself asking if I am a fraud and simply making a mountain out of a molehill. I can feel very guilty 'complaining' when others have died and others in the world, who are less privileged than me, are suffering the way they are. And yes, I have my life at this point and for that I am indeed grateful. It doesn't mean, however, that my life is at all easy or joyful. These conflicts within me make life even harder.

'My doctors and nurses may judge me'

I know many who suffer long term are wary of speaking out for fear of judgement and censure from their doctors, nurses and other healthcare professionals. They even fear that their care might be compromised if they speak out.

There are also those suffering long-term effects who do not even want to admit their problems to themselves. And I understand why. For example, fear of the cancer coming back in any form is terrifying, and not something most of us want to face. Furthermore, wanting life to be back to normal again is probably there in most of us. I also understand that it can be easier to keep our struggles to ourselves, even if we face them head on privately, in that we are then less likely to have to cope with others' judgement of us personally.

Also, most of us are told at the start of treatments that their effects will be limited. So from the onset, we are under pressure to experience and accept that version. As Katy, quoted in Macmillan Cancer Support's report about life after cancer treatment (2017), says, 'I think the expectation almost is, you have had cancer, you're over it, there's no more left, so therefore you're better. I felt that was the expectation and I tried to live up to it.'

Reason 4: Withholding and watering down information about treatment consequences

Privately, some doctors outside the oncology world, and occasionally even from within, have admitted to me that cancer treatments have plenty of nasty long-term effects that are not openly acknowledged but that are known about. One person who does acknowledge these effects is Dr Evans, who is featured later, in Chapter 7. Even though these doctors are very concerned about this issue, it can be extremely hard for them to speak out, not least because of their relationships with the drugs companies (see Dr Evan's comments later, in Chapter 7).

However, not telling patients and the world at large the whole story to date about what to expect from treatments for cancer, either shorter or longer term, militates against acceptance of them. If their existence is not acknowledged, it makes sense to say that when they appear, their existence will be a shock and possibly denied, both by those suffering them and those around them.

These days, doctors are actually required to flag up all the potential known side effects of treatment, and there are longer lists of potential problems on consent forms (Chan *et al.* 2017). However, there is still not enough transparency for some. As Olu, who had lung cancer three years ago, said,

> I had to ask over and over again what the risks would be. Some were mentioned, but I knew there would be others, and I met with a brick wall when I pushed to know and I ended up feeling like I was doing something wrong. In the end, I gave up, because I knew I had the cancer in my body and I just needed to get my surgery over and done with and hope for the best.

When you know you have cancer in you, as I know full well, it's true that you can't easily think about long-term effects, and any caring practitioner will be aware of this. All you want is to get the cancer out of you and to never have it again. Living on is the main concern, and it is a brave person who goes against medical advice and evidence and refuses treatment, or even part of it, for fear of long-term effects.

Nevertheless, many would argue that medical information before treatments start should always include clear, up-to-date data on their long-term effects, no matter how unsavoury they are – for example, there is an x percentage chance of this treatment causing sterility, lung cancer, sarcoma, etc. Some medical people might say that this is too brutal at such a hard time for their patients, so the truth needs to be watered down because it might put patients off the treatment they need. Others would argue that the brutal facts need to be disclosed.

'Acknowledging what we don't know is important, too'

Historically, it appears to be frowned upon in medicine to admit not knowing things. In fact, in general too, some might argue. However, sometimes no one knows what the risks are, and anyone diagnosed with cancer and facing treatment might well want to know this, too, or at least have a choice in the matter. There is much that medical science doesn't know.

However, a male colorectal cancer patient, quoted in Macmillan's report, *Throwing Light on the Consequences of Cancer and its Treatment* (2013b), confirms the need to give cancer patients truthful information and therefore real choices when he says, 'I had colorectal cancer. Its side effects affected my life badly. I should have been warned/advised about those side effects to decide. If I had known about them, I would not have gone ahead with surgery.' Easy to say in hindsight, you might say. Well, it depends on the relative risks each patient would be taking in refusing treatment or opting for less of it.

For my part, I am as certain as I can be that if I had had access to more of what was known at the time about the long-term effects of radiotherapy I would certainly have tried to insist on shorter courses, especially with my second cancer, which was less aggressive. As it is, I have been told several times that much of what I cope with physically now; for example, immune system problems, is very likely a result of the radiotherapies and other treatments I had. Despite my attempts prior to the treatment to ask about the longer-term risks, quite a lot that was known about was withheld, and the list of side effects listed on consent forms 15 years ago was much shorter than these days.

Reason 5: The 'unspeakables'

'It's hard to speak out about so-called "intimate" matters'

Many people who suffer the long-term effects of cancer have problems that are deemed 'unsavoury'. By 'unsavoury', I mean anything to do with bladder and bowel problems and problems with areas of our bodies that, in Western society, we do not easily speak about; for example, sexual organs and sexual function. The reticence to speak about these exacerbates the unspeakable nature of these long-term effects.

Furthermore, the impact of not speaking out is that it is then easier for those in healthcare and others to deny these effects, particularly since not everyone, even in healthcare, knows about their possibility or existence. Moreover, they are as susceptible as anyone else to feeling embarrassed talking about areas of our bodies that society has taught us to feel awkward about or ashamed of.

There have been many occasions when I have tried to talk to a doctor about muscular-skeletal pain, for example. When I have started to talk openly about my scars from breast cancer surgery, and explained that they run down one breast and across the other, an awkwardness and embarrassment has often interposed itself between us, presumably because I have said 'breast', an organ that is associated with sex in many societies. When, on occasion, I have tried to talk about how I feel about sex and body image since breast cancer, it is a rare person who does not flinch with awkwardness and/or embarrassment and want to change the subject.

'The need to speak out'

We need to talk more about these issues in order to encourage greater awareness and understanding, and help the many suffering with these 'unspeakable' but common problems. How we do that is a whole other matter. Professor Smith speaks about these matters in Chapter 7, and confirms that healthcare workers need to be more open with patients about so-called 'intimate' areas of the body. They also need to initiate conversations about symptoms, rather than waiting for the patient to do so, in order to improve the quality of life for those suffering long-term problems.

Reason 6: Collective attitudes to trauma

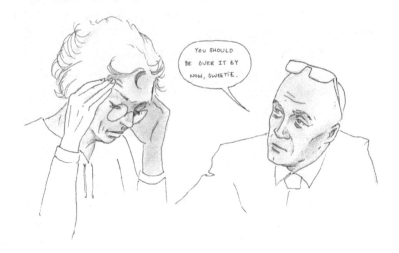

Received wisdom in many countries about how life is or should be after extreme trauma can easily colour how we view the thorny issue of the long-term effects of cancer. By 'we', I mean those affected, those close to those affected, those working with those affected and the world at large.

Most of us coping with extreme trauma, whether first or second hand, will tend to play down our thoughts, feelings and symptoms, telling ourselves they are not legitimate ones and that we are alone in feeling as extremely as we do. We might also tend to try to rationalise our reactions, but as Steve Haines says in his book on the subject (2016), we are not well equipped to rationalise trauma because, 'Most of the bits of the brain that deal with overwhelming events are very old. Some of the reflexes we use to respond to danger originated in reptiles.' This is a good point, yet little understood. We humans are not well wired when it comes to dealing with extreme trauma, be it cancer or anything else awful, in our complex world, and it is totally normal for us to be extremely discombobulated by it.

We know we're struggling like crazy, whether we are the person coping with cancer's aftermath or someone close to us, but we're also scared of speaking out because we have been conditioned not to, for fear of being considered 'unbalanced', 'mad' or 'over-reacting', etc. Most of us have been brought up in a society that has taught us, for example, that extreme emotional reactions to trauma are acceptable for a limited period of time. However, if they continue beyond that set period, usually about a year for a severe trauma, this is considered abnormal and the symptoms need to be treated, often with drugs such as antidepressants.

This conflict, between our raw, primeval responses to trauma and what we are told we should experience, can set up a huge tension in the minds of anyone who has deep and persisting emotions about cancer and how it has affected them in the long term, be they the ones with cancer or those close to them. Inside they are screaming, 'I'm still not coping with this. How can I be when I'm suffering these side effects/ when I'm watching them suffering/when my cancer can come back and/or get more aggressive at any point/when you are so scared someone close will get more cancer?' And this message we often get from others, that we are exaggerating our ongoing symptoms and that there is therefore something wrong with us psychologically, just heightens our suffering.

To add to the complexity of the situation, the net result of all this conflict can be that we can easily project some of this conflict onto partners, family, friends, patients, etc. As Raj, whose wife had breast cancer seven years ago, said,

> I just can't compute that my wife is still suffering so much. It seems to be getting worse. Her cancer isn't there anymore and yet she worries about it coming back. I know it can, but I put it to the back of my mind most of the time. Why can't she? I get really frustrated with her and lose my temper.

To be honest, I also know she isn't putting it on most of the time, but I don't understand it and I can't accept it and it makes us both unhappy. Bloody cancer. I hate it and I hate what it has done to us.

Reason 7: Misunderstanding the psychological impact of extreme trauma

'They just don't get how hard this is and they are making my life harder because of it'

I would argue vehemently, continuing on from my comments above, that many of us, including in the world of medicine and psychology, misunderstand how life naturally is for human beings after an extreme trauma such as cancer. Without meaning to we can easily become part of the problem for those coping in the long term with cancer, rather than the solution.

This happens when we confidently assert that those suffering long-term effects are 'making mountains out of molehills', 'putting it on', 'being over-dramatic', to name just three censorious opinions.

'Unpicking the process a little'

After any significant life trauma, in this instance, cancer and its aftermath, conventional wisdom usually asserts with vigorous and convinced authority that there will be a limit to the suffering. Furthermore, the suffering should be finished in no more than a year or two, or there is something seriously wrong. Progress should also be linear.

However, in both my clinical and personal experience, there is rarely, if ever, linear or limited progress through five stages, as trauma models such as Kübler Ross (still so influential and ingrained in our collective psyche) would largely assert there should be (Galgut 2012a, 2013b, 2014a). I have never heard anyone say they have progressed smoothly through all the stages, shock, disbelief, anger, etc., through to resolution and acceptance in about a year, including after a cancer diagnosis, its treatment and beyond.

However, as Caroline Lloyd in her book on demystifying trauma (2018) rightly says about bereavement, although her comments remain good for cancer,

> These models remain popular because they appeal to those who would like to impose structure on what can be an overwhelming emotional rollercoaster. They can also allow a bereaved person and those supporting them to feel as though they are in control, as if they can track their progress through a series of predictable stages. The reality of grief is that it can be unpredictable and uncontrollable. (Lloyd 2018: 36)

I can totally understand, in relation to cancer, how all concerned, from health professionals through to those coping with cancer, might find it easier to try to diminish and in a sense control emotional responses to this particular trauma for a variety of reasons, some highlighted in this chapter, also elsewhere in this book.

'Unfortunately, it appears we're not really wired that way'

Rather than admitting that long-term effects exist in ways that adversely affect people's lives, the easier stance is to time limit physical and emotional effects. Unfortunately, however, responses to having cancer are about as primeval as emotional responses can be, precisely because the nature of cancer is such that it knows no bounds, whether it appears to be contained or not. The possibility of more suffering and death is always just hovering overhead.

The uncontrollability of emotional reactions to trauma in general is undeniable, and many people experiencing trauma of all kinds have told me they don't experience much of what they are supposed to. For example, feeling shocked can come and go, or not appear to happen at all. Indeed, I remember well that when I was coping with my breast cancer diagnoses and treatments twice, in quick succession, I wasn't much aware that I was in shock. It wasn't until three or four years after my initial treatment ended that I started to feel the shock. It wasn't that I wasn't in shock at the start, I don't think; I just seemed to keep a lid on it, to get through all the awful things that were happening to me. I had to, otherwise I would have gone under.

Others have told me they felt likewise, and although there will be emotional impacts that are specific to individual cancers, there is also a clear commonality of experience too, not least the fact that emotions are non-verbal, unconscious physical responses and all humans experience them, whether we want to or not.

'Cancer surely can't be so traumatic or so never-ending'

Part of the misunderstanding in relation to the trauma of cancer and the existence of its enduring effects stems from continuing ignorance about how you don't just get diagnosed, treated and then recover. Even the luckier 'survivors' who have fewer side effects often take powerful medications for years and years after diagnosis that have profound medical consequences. I remember being really shocked myself by the unrelenting nature of treatments for breast cancer. I know other cancer treatments are often similar and can be worse. Indeed, some treatments last double the length of the ones I had, which lasted five years, and often enough the side effects don't go away and may get even worse, even though the treatments have ended. Of course, those with a secondary diagnosis of cancer usually have to endure tough treatments for the rest of their lives, a fact that many are not aware of or turn a blind eye to.

'Even the initial treatments are interminable. I don't think I can take any more. It's so stressful'

I hadn't realised how many stages there were to the initial phase after diagnosis: surgery, a long and complex several-staged process in itself, followed by radiotherapy, multi-staged and a long ordeal of six weeks, every day. I then had to cope with the whole process all over again, with a second diagnosis a few months after the first. After all this, I had to have adjuvant chemotherapy, as do most, in my case, four years of a large pellet being injected into the subcutaneous tissue of my abdomen, once a month, with a needle the width of a nappy pin. This caused me a lot of pain and extensive bruising, to say nothing of the horrible effects of having my ovaries switched on and off suddenly, several times, due to having to stop the drug twice, then restart it.

'It's all over. What's the problem now, then?'

It really did feel interminable, and I remember acutely how continuously battered I felt after all the intrusions and bad reactions I had, both skin-wise and systemically, even though I had finished all the treatments.

I remember trying to analyse the whole process in order to explain the enduring and cumulative emotional effects of the process to those who were incredulous when I said how I really was, and also in order to be able to describe it in a coherent way for my first book, *The Psychological Impact of Breast Cancer* (2010). In the end I came up with a diagram, which I have updated (see below) to include the additional impact of the long-term effects of cancer. This highlights how one trauma increases the impact of the next and is based on my experience of two diagnoses, two surgeries, two courses of radiotherapy spanning three months, daily, and four years of adjuvant chemotherapy, then the gradual appearance of long-term effects as time has passed. There has been no respite for me for the last 15 years, and I know others suffer like this, across a range of cancers, not just breast cancer. And yet it is a very rare person who says other than '15 years, that's amazing', which it clearly is. However, I hope I am making it abundantly clear that this is not the whole story.

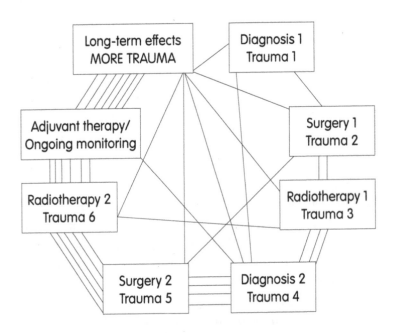

'The cumulative impact is not well understood'

To elaborate, the shock of, for example, surgery, is blurred into the shock of radiotherapy, increasing the trauma response still more and resulting in a build-up of stress, hence the increased number of lines as you progress from Diagnosis 1 through to long-term effects. There are so many shocks to deal with that the trauma of cancer becomes multi-layered and complex. All the lines criss-crossing on the diagram, linking one trauma to another, indicate this chaotic state of heightened stress.

Although not included in the diagram, other factors can make the complexity of the trauma response still more difficult. In the midst of coping, we can also be reminded of other traumas; for example, lying on a radiotherapy table, bare-breasted and being zapped with radiation can feel like a violation similar to sexual harassment or even sexual abuse, although clearly it is not. It may seem extreme to say this, but many of us, including myself, felt like this at points. And the unrelenting nature of even the shorter courses of radiotherapy that, in recent years, seem to be replacing the longer ones that I had, can easily contribute to a build-up of angst in anyone going through such an ordeal. It seems, and indeed it is, never-ending.

'Then, the impact of the long-term effects'

Dealing with the longer-term effects of cancer is also exposing those affected to constant re-traumatisation, and this is not well recognised. For example, any little symptom can induce panic that the cancer has come back, which, in turn, reminds us of the initial diagnosis and the trauma of that diagnosis.

'Do the effects really get worse over time? How can that be?'

At the point at which I was writing my first book, I hadn't properly realised that, for me, the physical side effects, and indeed the emotional ones, would, in a number of ways, get worse over time, not better. There was still hope in me that I would recover and get back to normal. And the message from the medics and healthcare people generally was, 'You're lucky, this was caught early'. At first, I was told I was cured, but that assertion changed, rightly so because breast cancer, no matter how small and contained, can recur at any time. That's one good reason why, when people say, 'You're alive, what's your problem?', this is an ignorant question, although clearly I am lucky to have survived to this point.

However, the quality of my life is pretty poor on more days than I care to admit to, most of the time (see Chapter 4). Getting over cancer just isn't a realistic hope for many of us. Fear of recurrence (see Chapter 3) is ever-present and in some ways worse, too, as I have more invested in surviving after all these years, hopefully free of cancer.

Reason 8: The pervading ideology concerning cancer's long-term effects takes no prisoners. It's a very scary beast to confront

As I end this chapter exploring some of the reasons why we tend to struggle to accept the long-term effects of cancer, and the fact that they pose problems for many, I want to stress, yet again, how hard it can be to challenge the dominant culture's entrenched position regarding these effects, both within healthcare and outside it.

'Self-doubt can get in the way'

Every time I pen a sentence for this book, I hear my external critic telling me I am talking nonsense. I also hear my internal critic. She tells me that my views are not valid enough, are over-stated and that I would do better to remain silent. It's tempting to do so, but, in the scheme of things, I am bold; many are not, and I understand why.

'Constant challenge is crucial'

The culture that exists in the healthcare world and outside it, that strongly resists acknowledging that these effects exist, needs constant challenging or nothing will ever change for the increasing numbers surviving cancer, many of whom understandably fear the consequences of speaking out.

Here, I rest my case, until Chapter 3 at least!

Summary

For those suffering the long-term effects of cancer:

- Trust your own experience and insights. You know better than anyone else what you are experiencing.
- You have a right to feel angry and to protest if your experience is being undermined by anyone, whether they are doctors, nurses, mental health professionals, colleagues, etc.
- It is normal to feel angry about having been diagnosed with cancer.
- It is normal to feel angry about suffering the long-term effects of cancer.
- It may help to challenge your own thinking about life after trauma. Cancer diagnoses and treatments are huge traumas, as are their consequences. It is not surprising if you feel emotionally bad, struggle to cope, etc., and the reality is that, as human beings, we are not wired to 'get over' and 'move on' through these traumas easily, or at all, in more cases than one might think.
- Unfortunately, the consequences of cancer can worsen over time. This happens to more people than we might

imagine, both emotionally and physically. It can help you emotionally to acknowledge this possibility, rather than deny it, although this might not be the right way forward for everyone (Galgut 2013c, 2016a).

- Feeling guilty because we have survived is common. We can also feel angry and resentful because our lives are hard.
- Many of us tend to play down our struggles with life post-cancer diagnosis and treatment. We have been taught to do so, and, obviously, nobody wants cancer to change their lives for the worse. However, it is a rare person for whom this is not the case, no matter what anyone or the media tells us.
- Unfortunately, life after cancer diagnosis and treatment is not well understood. It's probably worth remembering that not everyone will be unsympathetic; they are just unaware.
- Any educating of people you can bear to do will help us all. Equally, if you don't feel like doing this, that is fine too.

For healthcare professionals and others:

- Allow yourself to recognise that working with cancer patients with long-term effects can be very challenging. You're only human and subject to the same stresses, strains and emotions as the rest of us.
- It can pay dividends to question your own thoughts and beliefs about life after cancer diagnosis and treatment. For example, consider that the effects of cancer and its treatment can get worse over time, both emotionally and physically, rather than the reverse.
- Try to be honest with your patients about the side effects of treatments. Most people say they want this.

- Try to listen to what your patient is actually saying, even if you don't agree with them. Try to suspend your judgement a little. Most of us find this hard because of our entrenched thinking, but it can pay dividends if we can manage this, even to some small degree.
- Saying you don't know how they feel, but want to, can be validating of your patients.
- It can really help the patient in front of you if you are clear you believe that long-term effects exist. This validation alone can help them adjust to their situation.
- It can also help if you raise the subject, rather than leaving it to the patient – for example, 'I'm just wondering if anything has got worse over time, such as coping on a daily basis?'
- Raising the 'unspeakable' issues, if you can, may be a great help (see Chapter 7 for what Professor Smith says about this).
- Try not to put too much pressure on yourself to 'fix' things for your patients. This is probably unachievable anyway!
- Referring on to relevant colleagues, if and when necessary, can also be welcomed.
- Recognising your limitations, both to yourself and with your patients, can also help.
- It can be validating of your patients to admit that we are all human and that you are too.
- It is often just a validation of what they are going through, both physically and emotionally, that patients need and find supportive and useful.
- Remember that your patients often fear your judgement.

For family and friends:

- It can be helpful to challenge your own thinking about life after cancer if you are getting irritated with your partner or friend because they are not 'over' their cancer.
- Remind yourself that it is normal to be upset if your partner or friend is still suffering. You are only human and are entitled to support and understanding too.
- Try to suspend your judgement a little.
- Remind yourself that myths abound around the long-term effects of cancer, both emotional and physical. Many people don't just 'get over' cancer diagnosis and treatment.
- Offer your partner or friend a chance to tell you how they are and do your best to listen and not interrupt them. You could repeat back what they have said, just to check you have understood them.
- If your partner or friend is feeling strong enough, you could tell them how you feel and ask them to repeat what you have said back. Feeling heard can help both parties cope.

CHAPTER 3

DREAD OF GETTING MORE CANCER

A widespread and misunderstood long-term effect

Sod's law. Just as I was about to write this chapter, I developed a problem with my right leg. One morning, as I was walking around, it felt as though I had grazed my knee, which reminded me of how it felt when I scuffed my knees as a child. I didn't think anything of it, until I suddenly realised that I had a very large, hard swelling under my kneecap, near my shin. I was due to see a doctor, so I showed it to him and he sent me for an ultrasound immediately. This showed what might be a necrosis in the lymph node, probably nothing sinister, but there was some fluid around the area of the mass. Therefore, it was in the category of a suspicious lesion and possibly cancer. Anything to do with lymph nodes is particularly worrying for those of us who have had cancer already, as a problem with them can often enough herald unwelcome news of the cancer's return or spread.

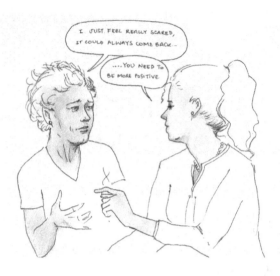

People don't understand why this dread haunts us so much. (Rumi, diagnosed five years ago)

It's hard to explain to anyone who hasn't experienced a cancer diagnosis what a terrifying situation this is. People often talk about cancer scares, which are awful in themselves, but for those of us who spend our lives being terrified of another primary diagnosis and/or the spread of cancer to other parts of the body, for example, bones or organs, or more metastases, it's a whole different ball game.

Although I am relatively fortunate in that, as yet, I have only had two primary diagnoses, I know I am not alone when I say that I can't imagine surrendering myself to more treatment for another cancer. The first two 'bouts' have left me with so many problems I can't imagine my psyche or my body coping with any more. Therefore, a situation such as the one described above, where I'm waiting to find out if the lump on my leg is more cancer or not, is nothing short of emotional agony, because it could effectively be the end of my life, imminently. And if there is one thing I fear more than death itself, it's having to live with the knowledge that I have an incurable cancer.

There are so many people living with incurable cancer and my heart goes out to them. I imagine you always have hope and indeed there are many people who live with incurable cancer for many years, but obviously it's a very different situation from the one I'm in.

I dread those words, 'you have more cancer'. Primary recurrence would clearly be less scary than spread to my bones and/or organs, but, obviously, I don't want to have to deal with either. The following may sound over-extreme to you, but the reality for me is that I often wonder whether I want to live on with that glinting sword of Damocles hanging over me all the time, blinding me, to varying degrees, on a daily basis.

You might find it hard to understand, but the two weeks I have just lived through, not being able to rid my thoughts of more cancer, were agony. Even though I had been reassured by a doctor I trust that he didn't think the lump was cancerous, he had still wanted me to have a repeat scan of it, to make sure it had reduced in size and the fluid had gone. During those two weeks I kept thinking, if he were 100 per cent certain it wasn't cancer, why would he want me to have a scan in two weeks' time? Was he keeping a 1 per cent chance it was cancer from me, to help me get through the two weeks? How could he have absolute knowledge, anyway? Was he just covering himself? Doctors have to, but I know him, and I didn't get that impression at all. I also kept thinking about the late effects of radiotherapy and about the things the oncologist, Dr Evans, had said when I interviewed him for this book, recorded in Chapter 7, about the possible late effects of radiotherapy in tissue that had received a low dose of radiation, namely, more cancer. These risks were small, but present.

Almost everyone I've ever talked to who's had a diagnosis of cancer says it's that tiny possibility that it might be cancer that haunts them. And we will carry that terror with us to our graves. Our imaginations run riot. Rational thought and weighing up percentage chances don't enter the frame during those times. It's just abject terror we experience.

A commonality of experience

People often say to me, well, we are all different, and that is a valid point, on many levels. However, I notice that there is a colossal commonality of experience when it comes to fear of recurrence and spread or worsening of a stable but still present cancer. I have talked to hundreds of people with a diagnosis of cancer over the years. Almost every one of them has admitted to this fear and terror, no matter how cautious they are about saying anything much about the impact of cancer on them in other ways. This is one thing that I can assert confidently and wholeheartedly, that 99.9 per cent of the people I have talked to agree on. The 0.1 per cent I don't include are the ones who say that their cancer is not going to come back, so they're fine. Maybe they are right to be so confident. I don't know. Some cancers certainly have lower recurrence rates than others.

Typical of what most people say, though, is Liz's comment. She had a malignant melanoma and says, 'I wake up in a cold sweat, thinking I have felt a lump and have to check.' Nightmares of this ilk are a regular occurrence for most of those who have talked to me openly about living with a diagnosis or recurrence of cancer.

Factors that make fear of recurrence and spread harder to live with

Others' lack of understanding and denial

The trouble with fear of recurrence is that this commonality of experience is just not recognised and understood and/or ignored, and equally so, the extremity of the fear. Additionally, the world at large often wants to mute this fear.

Medical people are no less susceptible to muting patients' extreme fear of recurrence than anyone else. I understand why, in that it is hard to sit with this degree of fear in a patient. It is also a taught belief that fear of recurrence will lessen over time, so medics usually really believe this.

I remember the oncologist who told me with great confidence that, over time, my fears would subside, and that I'd just feel the fear as I walked down the road on my way to my annual scan. The oncologist was very confident about this and not at all open to the idea that patients might mute how they felt for fear that their doctor might disagree and consider them to be 'over-reacting' or 'abnormal'.

Nor did the oncologist appear to question their stance in relation to fear of recurrence and whether it would increase over time. It didn't appear to enter their head that they might be wrong and that they could be causing patients extra emotional problems by asserting so assuredly that fear of recurrence always diminishes over time, rather than the reverse.

I also remember disagreeing with another oncologist, some years after diagnosis, because they couldn't understand my, what they considered to be, '"over-exaggerated" anxiety'. This oncologist's view was that I should be 'over cancer' by now and not worried about it coming back, because the chances were small. Easy for them to say, many of us would assert.

As I alluded to in Chapter 2, the problem is that medical people are seldom psychologically trained, and those who are, are usually very 'medical' in their understanding of human suffering; for example, psychiatrists. They, too, have been trained to accept a version of life post trauma that dictates that there is something psychologically wrong if the person is not over it in about a year. Few seem to question these beliefs, and, indeed, had I not lived through two breast cancer diagnoses myself, neither might I. Certainly, my training in psychology was very 'medical', the same views about life post trauma having been subscribed to.

Zena, diagnosed with ovarian cancer six years ago, speaks of a less than useful experience with a doctor when she says,

> I was referred to a psychiatrist a couple of years after my diagnosis, because I just couldn't shake off my depression about everything that had happened to me and how scared I was that the cancer would come back. The doctor I saw did seem concerned and was nice to me, but all he really had to offer was a diagnosis of depression, which wasn't news, and antidepressants. He didn't really get how I felt and I wondered if he thought I was overreacting because he kept going on about how I was going to be okay and that the passing of time would help. It still hasn't. I wish he had tried to understand my situation more and asked me more relevant questions.

Zena's experience is a salutary reminder to all of us in healthcare, maybe particularly in the arena of mental health, to try to question our entrenched attitudes, in this instance about fear or terror of recurrence, in case our practice runs counter to the needs of our patients.

'People don't want to know'

I do recognise that fear of recurrence and spread is a difficult issue for healthcare professionals and, indeed, society at large to understand, accept and want to know more about. As well as the entrenched beliefs about trauma, I think this also has to do with the fact that the extremity of the fear of recurrence and spread runs so counter to what we have been told is the right way to think about cancer, especially cancer that is contained.

These phrases, 'in remission' and 'got the all clear', are still so endemic in society and feed into the message that cancer is diagnosed, treated and usually cured or held at bay. So what's the problem? It's over and done with and there is no need to be scared. All is fine.

And, of course, as humans, most of us don't want to or haven't been encouraged to accept our terrors, not least of death, so our default position is not to do so. I can't remember how many times someone has pre-empted a conversation with me with, 'So you're all right now, are you?', meaning 'no more cancer, I hope', the subtext probably being, 'couldn't cope with that'. When I say, 'Not as far as I am aware', they almost always visibly relax, so presumably that is the subtext.

Strong emotions are hard to deal with

However, if I raise any tricky issues like, for example, 'my annual scan is coming up', and say, 'I'm very scared', a tension often interposes itself between us. Then, the response is either, 'Okay, I have to go', or 'Oh, you'll be okay', and they go on with what they want to say. If I express terror, it is usually clear that that is too much for others and that I am definitely over-reacting. And as I mentioned earlier, as a society, we tend to mute extreme emotion, not least because it is usually unacceptable to do otherwise. How many times have you heard someone say 'I'm a bit terrified' or suchlike, which is a contradiction in terms, really.

'You're making me feel worse'

There have sometimes been occasions when I have tried to engage openly and honestly with someone and have been told that my fears and suffering just make whoever I'm talking to feel worse about theirs. That's an interesting point, and it's true that if you, for example, feed back what someone is telling you, it can easily heighten their feelings about it, as I well know from my clinical work. Of course, when someone comes to therapy, more often than not they want validation of their feelings, whereas in everyday conversation, quite often people do not – at least, they don't want their feelings heightened. Sometimes, however, people will admit to being scared of getting cancer themselves. I totally understand and accept this fear and, of course, that fear is being constantly fuelled by, for example, the media.

It would be lovely if...

More people could cope with those of us suffering longer term from cancer and expressing how we feel, for example, about terror of recurrence. However, as the realist I am, I also know, of course, that you can't know how anything really feels in life until you experience it yourself, cancer included. And that creates an extra set of problems for all of us who suffer long-term with the effects of this appalling disease, not least, feeling isolated and marginalised.

I struggled to accept I was more frightened

My own ingrained beliefs that are a vestige of my training in psychology, as well as my upbringing, resulted in it taking a long time for me to realise that, contrary to conventional wisdom on the subject, I was becoming *more* scared of recurrence and spread as time went by, not less, as this wisdom predicts.

This realisation was a real revelation to me, and a shock. It was interesting and a relief that when I started to talk to others coping with cancer's effects, longer term, significant numbers of them confirmed that they, too, were more scared of recurrence with the passing of time. However, they also struggled to accept this fact because it was so contrary to the message we receive that the fear or terror will lessen. Nevertheless, as Sylvie, who was diagnosed with primary breast cancer five years ago, said, 'Until someone can tell me breast cancer doesn't ever come back, I'm going to be terrified that it will.'

In fact, breast cancer is one of those cancers that can come back, 30 years later, or at any point; it's just something those of us who have had the diagnosis have to live with. That common belief that people get the 'all clear' is a myth for many cancers, as far as I'm aware, and certainly for breast cancer, so that glinting and ever-menacing sword of Damocles is bound to loom large.

'I have more invested in not getting more cancer now'

As Frances, who was diagnosed with bowel cancer eight years ago, says,

> Immediately after the end of treatment, it can easily feel difficult to plan anything beyond the day itself. And any suggestion of a future can feel like an impossible thought, because it's hard to think in those terms. Even making any arrangements can feel too risky. As the weeks and months pass, the time frame begins to extend a bit. But even then, it takes a good long while to begin to believe you'll live on.

Like Frances and others, as time has passed, I am more able to believe that I might live on and therefore I have more invested in a future. I still rarely book anything much in advance, unless I really have to. And, of course, planning anything is difficult when you suffer all the physical long-term effects I endure, because I never know from one day to the next, one hour to the next, even, whether I'll be able to do those things, see those people, or not.

However, after 15 years, I dare to expect a scan to be free of cancer, not the reverse, and obviously I would much rather that than that more cancer is found.

Fear and dread of more treatment

This dread of more treatment, that I touched on earlier, is one that warrants expanding on as it can totally fuel a terror of recurrence. It's a really complex, multi-layered area to explore and what follows just scrapes its surface.

'So it's not just me, then'

It took me a while to realise that I was not alone in dreading more treatment, to the extent that I might decide not to have more and let the cancer run its course, if it comes back. Before ever having talked to fellow long-term sufferers about this, I had voiced my thoughts with a couple of my doctors. Both were horrified at the thought I might opt for no treatment and, therefore, death, over more treatment. 'Oh, no, you're too young', was one response. The idea that I might not fight to live on, even though I am only in my 60s, runs so counter to the mindset of the average doctor, who has been trained to save lives and not give up on patients, so I do sympathise. However, neither of them drew breath long enough to hear me out properly, and I have had to conclude that they just weren't willing or able to do so.

Listen more...

I do think the time has come for all of us in healthcare to listen more and better, even if what our patients are saying runs totally counter to our beliefs. As the patient, it was hard for me to talk to these doctors about how I felt about more treatment, especially since, yet again, I thought I was voicing something few people in my situation felt. I was both taken aback and relieved when someone said to me not long ago, when I was telling them how I felt, 'Well yes, I don't think I'd have more treatment, either.' Others coping with long-term effects have since said likewise when I have asked them directly, and I now believe it is a fairly common view. However, people are very reticent about speaking out about how they feel because:

- it runs so counter to what doctors and nurses expect us to say
- it sounds as though we are ungrateful for the life we have had since diagnosis
- it seems disrespectful of those who have lost their lives to cancer, their families and friends.

Treatments are still harsh

'But treatment surely isn't that bad, is it?', I've heard it said. Well, that's another taboo subject that I wrote about at length in my book *The Psychological Impact of Breast Cancer* (2010) and in my handbook *Emotional Support Through Breast Cancer* (2013a) from my own and others' perspectives, as well as in several articles that can be accessed via my websites.[1]

In brief, treatments for cancer are often still harsh, although plenty of doctors and others working in cancer care would probably hate to hear me say that. People want to think that things have improved, and in some ways, they have, but as far as I am aware existing treatments for cancer are basically the same as they were when I had them.

One myth is that chemotherapy is always worse than radiotherapy. As Lou, diagnosed 18 years ago with breast cancer, said,

---

1   See www.cordeliagalgut.co.uk and www.emotionalsupportthroughbreast cancer.co.uk

The chemotherapy made me feel pretty awful, tired, drained of all energy, but I was prepared for that and admit it wasn't as bad as I had thought it would be. I was less prepared for how bad the radiotherapy sessions made me feel. After the sessions, I would feel dizzy, my legs would feel as if they wouldn't hold me up and I felt nauseous. You don't generally hear that radiotherapy will make you feel ill and feel it should be a breeze.

To reiterate what I said in Chapter 2, I certainly found the two courses of radiotherapy and adjuvant chemotherapy I had physically and psychologically gruelling, so the thought of having more, even the shorter courses of today, and/or chemotherapy, fills me full of dread. My body has been battered enough, and I don't think I could cope with more, either shorter or longer term.

It comes down to individual choice and healthcare professionals respecting patients' choices. These treatments do appear to save lives – that's undeniable – and these days there can be treatment options that might be considered less harsh for example, immunotherapy, although from what I hear, these are gruelling, too. And they can have longer-term impacts.

The pros and cons of advances in treatment
A mixed blessing
Although treatments are more personalised than they used to be, as far as I am aware most people still receive a standard dose because that is the dose that has proven to be effective at killing the cancer, be it when treating with radiotherapy or chemotherapy. The problem is that as yet, nobody really knows what kind of dose each person will need to treat their particular cancer. In reality, some may actually not need any, others only a small dose, others the whole lot. Therefore, the state of play

being what it is currently, there will inevitably be those who are getting either treatment that their particular cancer possibly doesn't need or too much of it – over-treatment, effectively – potentially increasing the patient's risk of long-term effects. Dr Evans, in Chapter 7, talks about the problems of deciding how much treatment to give his patients. It's a hard decision, and not an easy position for any cancer doctor responsible for planning and treating a patient with cancer to be in.

As I understand it, some advances, for example, the Oncotype Dx test for breast tumours, also have pros and cons. To the extent that it is now much more possible to tell if a tumour is going to respond to treatment, e.g., chemotherapy, or recur by testing it in this relatively new way, obviously that's a great advance. However, had I been diagnosed recently rather than 15 years ago and had my first tumour been oncotyped (a very aggressive, albeit small, HER2+++ tumour, with no spread to either my lymph nodes or elsewhere in my body, including adjacent breast tissue), it could well have been that chemotherapy proper and/or Herceptin would have been recommended for me, because of the strong HER2 element, in spite of its contained nature. My oncologist wasn't really aware of HER2 tumours or their gradings, since the test was a relatively new one at that time.

In retrospect, the oncologist's lack of knowledge and the lack of an Oncotype Dx test were maybe a blessing. Chemotherapy proper, as opposed to the adjuvant sort that I had – which was horrible enough – on top of the two radiotherapies, could have left me even worse off today than I am. In fact, given the extremity of the burns I suffered from the radiotherapies and various other systemic effects, I honestly think full-blown chemotherapy treatment might have killed me. And the fact is that, despite the lack of these additional treatments, I am alive, 15 years after my first diagnosis. Furthermore, had I survived chemotherapy and taken Herceptin, although this drug clearly saves lives, its side effects can be many and potentially serious, so I am relieved I side-stepped that one, too.

I hope I am highlighting, as this chapter progresses, how fear of recurrence is complex and justifiable. Dread of more treatments and an enduring dearth of conclusive knowledge about their side effects, shorter and longer term, and of their effectiveness, significantly fuels this fear.

More complications

Lack of understanding of the terror that accompanies the thought of cancer coming back is further complicated by the fact that in the minds of the public, the media and those in healthcare, the cancer 'survivors' community gets crudely divided into those with a primary cancer diagnosis and those with secondaries (metastases). The primary diagnosis group is considered lucky, out the other side of cancer, back to normal, and unreasonable if they complain about their lot.

The secondary diagnosis group suffers an even worse deal – because there is spread of the original tumour, which has seeded elsewhere in the body – metastases, which clearly nobody would want. This group suffers an extra dose of people's ignorance and fear about their situation. Additionally, they are pitied and marginalised much more than the primary group, because, statistically, they are deemed to be nearer to death. And obviously, very sadly, this is probably so, although not certain.

However, and I take a deep breath before writing this, because what I am about to write is contentious and controversial within the cancer field and fairly taboo, the assumption that the lot of the person with a primary diagnosis is always better than that of a person with a secondary one can be erroneous. Indeed, I have talked to people with a secondary diagnosis whose cancer is thankfully controlled, who are not in constant pain and who have been stable for quite a number of years. Equally, I have talked to those with a primary diagnosis who suffer so much that they actually don't care if they live or die because their quality of life is so bad. Those are the extremes of both groups, you might say, to which I would respond, I'm not sure. It could be less polarised than that.

It goes without saying, however, that no reasonable, feeling person would argue that a primary diagnosis is worse than having metastases, for most people. All I am saying is that there might, often enough, be more crossovers between the two groups than we tend to assume.

Lack of understanding again

One thing is for sure and is worth reiterating. Both groups are not well understood by many of those in healthcare, in the UK and elsewhere. There are few listening ears for either group, and the physical and emotional needs of both groups are currently simply not being adequately met. Given that there will soon be an epidemic of people who are surviving cancer and suffering its long-term effects, I'm really not sure where that leaves us all, except to start raising more awareness of these issues as soon as possible.

Dread of recurrence and spread is so complex

Indubitably, there is much more seething beneath the surface for those of us terrified of recurrence than might at first be apparent. I hope that I have conveyed that, at least, in this chapter.

Summary

For those suffering the long-term effects of cancer, remember that:

- There is a universal fear of recurrence and spread, whether others say so openly or not.
- Fear and terror of check-ups or scans, etc. is perfectly normal and to be expected.
- If you talk to someone else who has had cancer and they say they're fine, it's possible they are, but it could also be their way of coping with their fear and terror.
- You are definitely not alone if you suffer fear and terror about your cancer returning or getting worse, so don't let anyone tell you differently. It's actually a normal emotional response, as a human being, to feel this fear and terror.
- It also makes sense that we might fear recurrence more as time goes by.
- There is no right way to feel. If you are not aware of fear and terror, that is fine, too.
- Doctors, nurses, our families, friends, work colleagues, etc. are often not psychologically trained. Healthcare providers are, therefore, as likely to have the same misconceptions about how we feel as society at large.
- It is totally normal to fear more treatment and to doubt whether you would consent to more. Some people will be unsure or fear it but have it anyway, and some might refuse. Both choices are valid.
- The choice about whether you submit to more treatment is, many would argue, yours alone, and not your doctors', nurses', partners', children's, etc. decision.
- It can help to tell yourself, out loud, that you are allowed to feel the way you do, no matter what anyone else tells you to think and feel. Start with, 'I am allowed to feel'...and continue as you choose.
- You are still allowed to complain, even if you have a good prognosis, and expect your feelings to be heard and accepted.

- If you're struggling with a secondary diagnosis, you're allowed to say what you like about it and expect to be accepted and attempts made to understand your position and your needs. You have a total right to accept nothing less.

For doctors, nurses, etc.:

- It will help your patients if you can suspend your judgement as best you can as to how they feel about fear of recurrence and spread, fear of more treatment, etc.
- Take the time to listen. Not being psychologically trained doesn't mean you can't help. Simple phrases such as the following can help more than you could possibly imagine:
  - 'This is new to me – I want to know.'
  - 'I have heard what you said.'
  - 'I want to help as best I can.'

Remember that it's okay to say you are not psychologically trained and that you need to refer on – you can't do everything. It is also okay to admit you don't know something. Your patients might well appreciate you admitting this.

For family and friends:

- It can be hard to accept that your partner/family member/friend's fear of recurrence doesn't dissipate.
- It's only natural to want partners/family/friends to have recovered from cancer.
- You will naturally worry that your partner/family/ friend is going to get more cancer.
- It can be hard if both you/your partner/family member/ friend are all worrying about the cancer returning.
- Expressing how each of you feels can help. You could encourage your partner/family member/friend to tell

you how they feel and reassure them you won't judge them and will listen.

- You could then feed back what you have heard to them.
- You could ask them if they are okay with you saying how you feel too, checking out they have heard you correctly.

The following section may be of interest if you are wondering what the benefits of emotional support with a trained professional might be and how to go about finding someone.

The benefits of counselling or psychotherapy for those suffering the long-term effects of cancer

There are many benefits, in my opinion, providing you can access a psychologist, counsellor or psychotherapist who is a good fit for you. Obviously, this is not so easy if you are not able to pay for one privately, although you can be referred through your GP and you do have a degree of choice (in the UK at least). There are so many different kinds of therapists and theoretical approaches. The best way to understand the differences is to look on one of the websites listed at the end of this section.

Broadly speaking, psychologists have to be registered with the Health and Care Professions Council (HCPC). Our title is protected, and these days, we need to be trained to doctorate level, so you know that if you see a counselling or clinical psychologist, we are mostly trained to that level. This doesn't mean that you will get on with every psychologist, however.

There are also many counsellors and psychotherapists you could see and many are well trained. There are senior accredited and registered counsellors or psychotherapists who have a lot of clinical experience and also those who have less, so it is important to check qualifications and experience before agreeing to see someone.

I use the terms 'counsellor', 'psychotherapist' and 'therapist' interchangeably. All three work shorter and longer term with clients, as do psychologists, and the only way to be sure what any counsellor, psychotherapist or psychologist offers is to check out their details on an individual basis.

Therapists' experience of supporting people with long-term effects

Regarding the issue of the long-term effects of cancer, you could ask any potential counselling or clinical psychologist, counsellor or psychotherapist if they have any experience of working with people living with cancer's long-term effects. There are some organisations that clearly do have experience in the field. They may or may not be right for you. The only way to know is to speak to therapists working for them or go and see them for a one-off session and decide for yourself.

Some therapists without experience of people with cancer might still be of use; it just depends. Unfortunately, my profession mirrors the world at large on this issue. You might say, well, they should be more understanding and accepting than the world at large, and I would agree. Hopefully, this is generally so, although I'm afraid it's not always the case.

'This doesn't feel right'

If you find yourself in a session with someone who isn't understanding you and your situation, you have a complete right to say so and to waste no more of your time and probably your money, too. You could say, 'I'm sorry, but I'm not feeling understood and accepted enough', or words to that effect. If the therapist responds with something along the lines of, 'I want to. Tell me how I'm not doing that for you', that's a good sign.

However, I would suggest you go with your gut instinct as to whether you stay or leave.

Unfortunately, a therapist who has had cancer is not always the right choice either. If they disclose that they have had cancer, this can be helpful. If they talk about their experience a lot and 'miss' yours, that's usually not helpful, although disclosing they have 'insider knowledge' of cancer can really help. Even disclosing some experiences they have had can be helpful, providing this doesn't get in the way of the fact that it's your therapy and not theirs. Again, ultimately, you have a total right to leave the relationship. There are plenty of good therapists around in most cities in the world, if you want face-to-face sessions. And, of course, many of us work online now, so the choice is far greater.

Therapy, cancer and me

Having written the paragraphs above, I can't say I have found the ideal therapist to support me with the long-term effects of cancer (Galgut 2011, 2014b). Personally, I would never see a therapist who hadn't had a lot of therapy themselves – I think you need to understand how it feels to be a client as well as a therapist.

Therefore, I still have therapy periodically to make sure I get support with my personal issues, as part of ongoing self-development work. This is a requirement of my registrations and accreditations, and an initiative I totally support. I have used my time with my therapists, over the years, to support me through cancer, particularly during the first few years.

Validation of how I was feeling was key. I did have a therapist who had had cancer, so she understood what it was like to be on the other side of the cancer fence. That was very helpful. But since the long-term effects kicked in, I haven't really found a therapist who 'gets it'. I'm about to try again with a new therapist, so we will see.

To be honest, providing the therapist listens, seems to understand well enough and allows me to offload, that'll be fine. If they start trying to tell me how I should think and feel, I'll be out of the door as fast as my legs can carry me. For me, personally, unless my therapist can offer me a way of looking at my situation that is new to me, is helpful and non-judgemental, I'm better not expecting too much. That way, I'll get more from the experience. I think I have a duty to be clear about what I want from my therapist, however. In my case, it is just a chance to offload, in a safe space, away from my everyday life, with someone who doesn't know anyone in my life.

A therapist who has had cancer or not?

For me, the ideal therapist is one who can suspend their judgement as much as possible, listen and show they understand what I am presenting well enough. These days that is more important to me than anything else. I also need them to be clear about whether they have had cancer or not and what their experience of cancer is if I'm going to them for support with anything related to cancer. For example, has a family member/friend of theirs had cancer/died, etc.? I need them to be able to say they don't know something when they don't, rather than pretending. Therapists might well be reticent about answering some of these questions, and the whole issue of therapist self-disclosure is a contentious one in my profession. However, it is a live issue these days, and it is reasonable to expect this kind of openness from a therapist.

I'm aware that I am a tough client, after all my years of therapy, clinical practice and thinking about all these issues a lot. Anyone reading this book might be thinking I am being too exacting, but as I say above, I am describing my ideal therapist.

Most of us, including me, don't match up to that very often, and that is fine, since we are all human.

Counselling and psychotherapy organisations

Although the following are UK-based organisations, there are similar ones in other English-speaking countries as well as in other non-English speaking countries across the world. It is also easy to search on the internet and find therapists across the world.

British Association for Behavioural & Cognitive Psychotherapies (BABCP)
www.babcp.com

British Association for Counselling and Psychotherapy (BACP)
www.bacp.co.uk

British Psychological Society (BPS)
www.bps.org.uk

United Kingdom Council for Psychotherapy (UKCP)
www.psychotherapy.org.uk

Questions you might want to ask a potential therapist

It can be very hard to ask a potential therapist any of the questions below. You could email them, if you prefer.

- What are their qualifications? You may want to see proof of these and of their registrations and accreditations. Many therapists have websites with these listed and professional websites they can refer you to, to check their registrations and accreditations.
- How much experience do they have of seeing clients?

- Do they have particular specialisms?
- Do they routinely support people coping with cancer's long-term effects?
- How do they feel about the topic?

Any question that is important to you is okay to ask, although a therapist is within their rights to refuse to answer a question. However, if they refuse you have a right to ask them why they have refused. You can then make a decision, based on their overall responses. Other issues regarding how they work, prices, etc., should be available either on their website or listed somewhere. If not, ask them.

Email them if you prefer. Hearing someone's voice can be useful, too, so you could ask to have a short chat with them, if you are satisfied with their email responses. If your gut tells you they are not right for you, have the confidence to move on to the next therapist. There are plenty of us around! It is a competitive market and many of us will want to help.

CHAPTER 4

MORE LONG-TERM EFFECTS, PHYSICAL AND EMOTIONAL

I was incredulous

If someone had told me, 15 years ago, when I was so new to breast cancer, that I would still be suffering its effects years later, I would have found that very hard to believe. Everything I was being told contradicted that notion. In fact, I remember several doctors telling me that it would be downhill all the way after surgery and radiotherapy, and I didn't really doubt them for a moment. This was partly because I wanted to believe that that would be so, and partly because it wouldn't really have occurred to me that they might be wrong. They were the cancer specialists after all.

I wanted to believe my doctors

I also needed to believe my doctors during such a terrible time, and conventional wisdom says that doctors know best. Despite the fact that a doctor at the time had told me emphatically that I didn't have breast cancer (as I was too young), when, in fact, I did, I still retained a somewhat blind faith that doctors knew better than I did what might ail me physically. This faith in medical doctors, although somewhat shaken, remained intact for a little while with the cancer doctors I met, even after a bad experience with my first breast surgeon. At that point I also had an oncologist I liked and trusted.

My trust then disappeared

However, most of my trust in their clinical judgement, and even more so in the breast surgeon, was swiftly erased on the day I received my second diagnosis; it was never to return. In fact, many years later I am still haunted by the mistakes that were made (see below), including the fact that the oncologist dismissed my strong belief I had cancer in the other breast. The oncologist did, at least, send me for a scan, but made it clear they thought my fears were the result of an overactive imagination and told me to go away for a week before I had the scan, which I did.

Furthermore, on that 'Diagnosis 2' day, the radiologist didn't believe there was a tumour in my left breast. They knew I had had one diagnosed in my right breast a few months earlier, so presumably they thought this lessened the chances of another. The mammogram they did was clear, in their view, and they wanted to send me away without ultrasounding the breast in question. However, I insisted they did so, much as I wanted to run away. In a disgruntled mood, they agreed. I showed them where I thought the tumour was, and lo and behold, they were able to see it quite clearly. They looked incredulous, but it was impossible to deny. This breast hadn't previously been ultrasounded – they didn't routinely ultrasound women's breasts as well as mammogram them. The tumour was 1.5 cm, so would almost certainly have been visible on ultrasound at 'Diagnosis 1'. This gross negligence could have cost me my life.

Being assertive saved my life

It was my intuition plus my assertiveness with doctors that very likely saved my life; my insistence that the GP refer me, my insistence that the oncologist listen to me and my insistence that the radiologist ultrasound an area of my breast they believed didn't need ultrasounding. It wasn't easy being that assertive with such experienced doctors, several times over, but thank goodness I was. I might well have been dead if I hadn't.

'You're imagining it'

Sadly, I am as sure as I can be that none of these doctors would believe the reality of my current situation. I think they would either put most of my symptoms down to generalised hysteria, and/or assert that they were not related to cancer treatment in any way.

A legacy of distrust 15 years on

Although I would say that a distrust of all of us in healthcare and a questioning stance are preferable, and even necessary, for anyone negotiating a cancer diagnosis, shorter and longer term, I think I have been left with an understandable excess of both. I have lost count of the number of times I have been told that I am over-anxious, over-vigilant, too clever for my own good and suchlike. As a consequence, the lesson I have had reinforced repeatedly is that the complacent attitudes that are too often present in UK healthcare, can and do result in a blinkered approach. This, in turn, can have serious consequences for patients on the receiving end of these attitudes if left unchecked.

Listen and learn

There is the doctor, for example, who cannot entertain the thought that there might be another tumour in their patient's breast because they trust their colleague who referred the patient on to them. And I have a certain sympathy for a doctor in this predicament – you can't be doubting colleagues' clinical judgements all the time or you'd go insane. However, when you have a patient telling you their instinct tells them something is wrong, points to an area on their body they are worried about and does so repeatedly, it is surely time to listen and hear, and not to dismiss.

Then there is the medical doctor, with no training in psychology, for whom I have little sympathy, who pronounces their patient over-anxious and wrong when they say they are still suffering the effects of treatment for cancer. They refuse to listen and refuse to accept that which is not to their liking, even if there is empirical evidence available and they have adequate evidence right in front of their noses.

'I'm laughing to myself'

I'm chuckling to myself as I write this, because I can hear the voices of my critics in healthcare, some of my colleagues, in effect pronouncing me 'unreasonable' for still suffering from this legacy of distrust. I can just hear them saying, 'Oh, there she goes again. So many unresolved issues, unresolved anger, inability to trust doctors and lay the past to rest.' And I'd have to agree with the 'feeling angry' bit because it's palpable as I read these paragraphs back.

Belittling in order to bolster

The fact that I have had many years of training in psychology and related disciplines, and so many years' clinical experience, counts for absolutely nothing with these particular people. I am 'just' a patient when talking about cancer's psychological effects on me, whether I do so from my dual perspective or not.

I want to make it clear that I have met a good number of healthcare professionals who are much more aware and reflective than those mentioned above, so I'm not talking about *all* health professionals. Nevertheless, those I refer to above are often influential, the bastions of the establishment, whose tactics are sadly to belittle in order to bolster their often outmoded practices and beliefs.

So where does that leave the person who is struggling with long-term effects?

As I well know, it is possible to feel extremely alone and desperate. Macmillan Cancer Support's report, *Am I Meant to Be Okay Now?* (2017), is full of examples of people who have been extremely thrown by how different the reality of their lives is from that which they were led to expect. But even this report doesn't include anyone suffering years after cancer, for example, 10 years plus. No doubt those involved in producing this report know that it's hard enough to get healthcare professionals and society at large to accept the problems that exist two years after diagnosis let alone 10 or more years on from diagnosis.

Since diagnosis in 2004 and beyond

I've just found an article I wrote as recently as 2016, in the British Association for Counselling and Psychotherapy journal, *Private Practice*, which was shocking for me to read because I was so physically and emotionally low when I wrote it. Currently, I'm differently challenged, I would say. I will expand on this statement in what follows, but I think it would be interesting to share a bit of that 2016 article with you, entitled, 'Survived, but at what cost' (Galgut 2016b). I borrowed this title, in part, from Macmillan's report of a similar name (Macmillan Cancer Support 2013a), which highlighted that life is often enough not all a bed of roses after surviving cancer – a contentious, but pertinent, report when it came out. And it still is.

Prior to 2016, so for the 12 years that I had survived post diagnosis and cancer treatment, I documented the problems, both emotional and physical, that I encountered, in various things I wrote; for example, in my books and in a number of articles (Galgut 2010, 2012b, 2013d, 2014a, 2016c). In these writings I described the same degree of physical upset and emotional desperation that is so obvious in the excerpt below, complicated by the impact of my mother's death on me.

However, the sheer exhaustion of the cumulative effect of all this suffering, and my rawness, is particularly stark. I wrote this partly while in hospital, on and off, for several weeks. The intrusion of constant cannula replacements, infusions, blood tests, blood pressure readings, scans, etc., had really taken their toll, in addition to feeling so ill from the sepses. These intrusions, although clearly necessary, are much harder to tolerate now, due to scar tissue, pain and risk of infection. I had had enough.

....

I'm writing this article from my hospital bed, having been admitted with a second sepsis in a month. The only explanation the doctors can give for this turn of events is the long-term effects of cancer treatment, specifically radiotherapy, which appears to have adversely affected my immune function.

To say that I'm at the end of my tether both emotionally and physically is a big understatement. In fact, I feel desperate about both my immediate situation and the future, not helped by society's general lack of awareness of long-term effects. More understanding would help me in my situation, both emotionally and maybe even medically. Interestingly, when I asked the consultant, 'Do you think these sepses could suddenly kick in 12 years after breast cancer diagnosis and treatment?' he replied in the affirmative. 'I've seen this before', he said. I've heard this before from other medical people as well. The more I coax information out of them, the more I hear confirmation that they have groups of patients whose clinical picture is similar to mine. As mental health professionals, I wonder if we're sufficiently aware of these possible long-term effects and the impact on those of us affected, both clients and colleagues. Perhaps not, since there's so little publicity about them.

I've written before in BACP journals and elsewhere about the effects of cancer treatment on me longer term, but this article is a step on from these – a more desperate me writing this time. I'm not sure that I've ever written in such an immediately raw way. Life is currently so bleak for me, dominated by sepses and other less extreme infections. In between, the quality of my life is not at all good. Symptoms range from 'liveable with' to 'impossible', depending on how unwell I am. Regular dizziness and muscular-skeletal problems limit my activity. I'm basically an active person who loves life, when well, am interested in lots of things and I like to travel. For the last few years, if in the average day I can get through it feeling relatively OK, that's a good day for me. I travel by watching relevant programmes on the television and take pleasure in as much as I can; the robin on the window sill, the scent of lilac in the garden at dusk, the hue of the sky and trees in different lights.

And yet, there are more days than I care to admit to when I think life isn't worth living. I don't want to end my life, I just want it to be better. People say, 'You're lucky you survived, such and such a person died.' And it's true. Victoria Wood's death from cancer was a big shock recently. I felt so sorry for her, her children, anyone who loved her. I've recently turned 61, so we were pretty much of an age. I know I'm lucky, I still have life and a degree of hope, but my life is in shambles, currently, and hope is waning fast. It's a very depressing situation and I get very low, coping with the general lack of awareness about the long-term effects of cancer treatment.

Now

Currently, apart from the fear of recurrence, I am not feeling quite as emotionally raw. I think it is possible that some of the rawness was a byproduct of constant infections and regular sepses. It's a little different now, in that the excellent urogynaecologist I have has managed to improve my quality of life to some degree, by sticking with me and suggesting different strategies and drugs, to reduce the back-to-back urinary tract infections I was suffering from. For example, I'm now taking an anti-inflammatory drug that sometimes helps, and so far this year I have only been in hospital once.

It helps to get possible explanations

I have recently been told that the cancer treatments I had were probably responsible for the heavily inflamed bladder I have had since treatment, which had huge numbers of mast cells present when a piece of tissue from it was examined under the microscope a couple of years ago. There is also much mast cell activity in other parts of my body; for example, in my upper and lower digestive tracts, as recent biopsies have revealed. At this point in time, no one can be absolutely sure why, but it helps me just to know that cancer treatment could have caused much of this. I wonder how many others are in the same or a similar predicament, diagnosed or not?

Critics would no doubt say, well, at a pinch, after radio-therapy to the breast and the chest wall, maybe an ongoing inflammatory response is explicable in that immediate area, but not in the bladder, or throughout the digestive system. However, I have been told by less sceptical medical people that radiotherapy's immediate and longer-term effects can be systemic, no matter which area of the body is treated, so the bladder could be affected. I actually remember complaining of a systemic response, dizziness, nausea and general malaise during both radiotherapy treatments, and had my first full-blown urinary tract infection then, too. These effects were mostly dismissed or underplayed by the doctors and nurses looking after me at the time. Nevertheless, I remember others going through radiotherapy complaining similarly. Dr Evans' comments in Chapter 7 throw some light on what might be happening to me and to others like me, as do Professor Smith's in the same chapter.

Other ongoing bug bears

I also continue to struggle with vestibular problems, caused by worsened migraine, possibly exacerbated by cancer treatments, plus the inflammatory responses mentioned above, and additionally, benign positional vertigo. These vestibular problems, that cause, namely, dizziness, nausea, malaise, visual disturbance, perception problems, among other symptoms, continue to dominate my life on a daily basis. As I mentioned earlier, they all started during my first radiotherapy, except for the migraine. So perhaps it makes sense to suggest that they might be related to that assault on my body and were exacerbated by the second course of radiotherapy I had after the second diagnosis, and no doubt the four years of adjuvant chemotherapy too. Some medical people also hypothesise that cancer itself can cause negative longer-term effects that are not a recurrence but a byproduct of the body dealing with the disease. This is an interesting idea.

'Get a life; it'll do you good'

Yes, I have been instructed to do this. And yes, it does upset and anger me when people say these things and it feels very unfair, not least because I try hard to have a life. However, going out and about is a veritable obstacle course of potential problems, and there are times when I just can't face it. I can fall – not wise with osteoporosis, a condition caused and exacerbated by the adjuvant chemotherapy drug. I can panic, literally, because the objects around me appear bigger or smaller than they are or they appear to move. This is due to the malfunctioning of my vestibular system, I am told. The net result is that a journey from A to B on foot or in a moving vehicle can be like a nightmare version of a ride on a Big Dipper, which some might say is already enough of a nightmare experience.

However, I try not to stay indoors too much because then I feel housebound. Crowds can make me panic, though. I might get mowed down, since few people seem to step aside these days, and I am unsteady on my feet. I'm remembering something that happened a while back. I was going up the escalator in a favourite department store of mine and I started to panic, seemingly for no good reason. I was on my way to buy something, I was happy about that, but I had to leave because I started to feel so bad. It went through my head that it was my beloved mother, from her grave, stopping me from spending money, since she never approved of me doing that. This made me smile, but I realised there were other reasons, of course. However, it wasn't until I spoke to my doctor who specialises in vestibular problems that I understood that the lights in the shop, the movements around me, and suchlike, had very likely overloaded my system and had caused the panic.

It's hard to overstate how much this continuation of problems adversely affects my life. It's often impossible to have any social life, since these problems are constant. Although on some days they are less intrusive, mostly they are intrusive. Therefore, if I have, for example, arranged to meet someone, I can either turn up and quite likely feel terrible, which impacts on them, or I can cancel, which also impacts on them. Sometimes people understand, and sometimes they don't. Either way, it's miserable for me, and these problems affect every area of my life, such as my work (see Chapter 6).

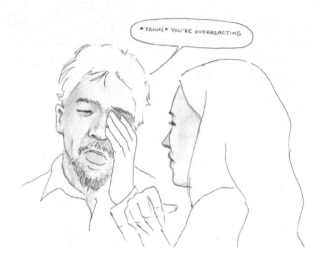

'You must be exaggerating'

I know muscular-skeletal problems are common, especially as we age. Many of us have them and not just those of us who have had cancer. However, the sort I have literally paralyse me often enough, and severely affect my mobility a lot of the time. Most of those I know with the usual sort of age-related problems manage to get on with their lives, socialise, go on holiday, etc. For me, even walking can be hard, and it's always painful to varying degrees. Today, for example, I am limping around, unable to move much at all. I find this so frustrating and soul destroying. And I never know when I am going to have a better day or not. The scar tissue I have gets very tight. Some in healthcare believe that radiotherapy affects the ability of tissue to repair itself, in the long term. Presumably this can contribute to the tethering of skin and associated nerve pain I suffer from. I have also developed inflammatory conditions all over my body, which some assert are cancer treatment-related, for example, bursitis.

It is a great physical ordeal writing this book, for example. This is because the movement in my writing/typing arm/s is severely affected by, for example, scar tissue and the breaks to both that I sustained a few years ago. The pain when I write/type is difficult to cope with. It radiates down my body and because I am dizzy, my body stiffens up as my brain tries to keep me upright rather than toppling over. That exacerbates the problem.

I am determined to keep going, though. The one thing that might stop me is if I get repeated sympathetic nervous system activation from inflamed nerves or tissue, tethered scar tissue issues, etc. This makes me very unwell until it subsides. I'm a very determined person, but this stops me in my tracks. Movements that used to be simple ones are huge mountains to climb now. Anything that requires my arms is problematic. The same often applies to my legs and feet. Stirring, pulling, pushing, reaching out, stretching, etc., are often so painful – and cause cramps and spasms – that I give up. I really enjoy cooking, and many other activities that involve these movements, so these problems are extremely annoying, frustrating and depressing. Thank goodness for my physiotherapist, who is the only one whose treatments afford me some relief.

'This can't be radiotherapy – that's not possible'

As I have said, in many circles the whole phenomenon of the long-term effects of radiotherapy is contentious. I've outlined some of the issues that might well be related above. Unfortunately, however, there are more. It's always hard talking about 'radiotherapy scatter', which is when some of the radiation used within the treatment field travels beyond it, to adjacent tissue. For example, beneath both my breasts, and spreading right down my torso, there are big brown mole-like things and other unsightly growths that have grown and changed over time. I have been told these are 'scatter' from radiation and they have certainly appeared since the treatment and look related. Although superficial, they definitely have an effect on my self-esteem, which I expand on a little in Chapter 5.

However, more concerning from my point of view is how the organs beneath the scatter have been affected by the two radiotherapies and possibly the adjuvant chemotherapy. There is some evidence of this in, for example, my liver and digestive system, and I live in constant fear of radiotherapy-related cancer, the risk of which increases, rather than diminishes, over time; for example, lung cancer, oesophageal cancer, blood cancers and blood vessel cancers (see Dr Evans' comments in Chapter 7).

Trauma upon trauma

I have often relied on my partner of 37 years to help me practically, especially since diagnosis, but she is now 70. She is also not in great health, having recently been diagnosed with dementia. This has catapulted us both into a state of panic; one more trauma to bear, on top of cancer's fall-out, increasing the stress response, in much the way that I referred to in Chapter 2.

I know I will be limited in how much I can help her practically, as she gets even worse. This worries me all the time, and also whether my own cognition will remain intact. Although, thank goodness, I can currently think for both of us, I can't stand or sit for long. Driving is very hard for me, and my partner can't drive any more. Public transport is also very hard to negotiate. I can hardly believe we have ended up like this. How many others are in this predicament, coping with the fall-out of cancer on top of other serious problems? Plenty, I imagine.

I could really do without cancer's fall-out, for us both. However, I'm stuck with it, and my job of work is, I fear, to make the best of it and to value what I have as best I can, allowing myself to rant and rave as much as I need to. Who knows what the future holds. Tomorrow, next week, next year – recurrence, spread, worsened effects. Maybe some improvement... The latter would be wonderful, but I suspect the former possibilities are more likely... And on I go...[1]

Summary

Overall, it can really help those suffering longer-term if health-care workers, as well as partners, family and friends, can offer some understanding and practical support. Even a few kind, understanding phrases or questions, such as the ones that follow, can really help:

- 'It must be so hard for you.'
- 'You must get so fed up.'
- 'What can I do to help?' (It doesn't have to be much – even a small gesture will very likely be appreciated.)
- 'I understand, as best I can, how hard your life is.'

For those of us coping with the kinds of problems outlined above, Deirdre King, an autogenic therapist, suggests ways we can support ourselves that might be of use. Indeed, anyone living with or working with those coping longer-term with cancer might also find these strategies useful.

---

1 For more examples of the long-term effects, please see Mitzi Blennerhassett's testimony, in the Appendix at the end of this book. She had both anal and breast cancer, and is author of *Nothing Personal: Disturbing Undercurrents in Cancer Care* (2008), which won the Medical Journalists' Open Book Award in 2009.

Switching off your fight or flight response

Deirdre suggests that the following body scan may be helpful. Ongoing stress keeps the fight–flight response switched on for long periods, causing further stress. Relaxing switches on the rest and recuperate response, which allows your body to repair itself. If you feel comfortable connecting to your body, try this body scan:

- Find a quiet place where you will not be disturbed. You might like to shake surface tension out of your body first and take a couple of deep breaths. Sit or lie comfortably and close your eyes.
- Take your attention to your body and gently scan either up or down it for a few minutes. Notice how you feel and any physical sensations, the pulses and rhythms of your body. No need to try and change what you observe. Accept it, without judgement or criticism, as what is going on for you right now.
- Let your breathing do what it does naturally as you quietly observe.
- At the end of your body scan, yawn, stretch and open your eyes. Get up slowly.

Deirdre says, if emotions come up, try to acknowledge them and let them be.

You could also try the following offloading exercise to relate to your emotions, but leave an hour before and after doing a body scan.

If you do want to release feelings that you think have got stuck, you could also try the following: this exercise, based on an Intentional Offloading Exercise from autogenic therapy, helps to release feelings that have got 'stuck'. It is not necessary to actually feel the feelings while you do this exercise, although it's fine if you do.

- First decide what you want to work on – for instance, you could work on your sense of shock and panic. Find a place where you will not be interrupted to do your exercise. It is best not to do it an hour or so before going to bed. Always work within your comfort zone, stopping if you feel uncomfortable.
- Take a single phrase that strongly expresses how you feel. Repeat the phrase out loud over and over again until you come to a natural stop or the phrase becomes mumbling. For instance, you might say 'I'm scared' or 'I'm furious with people belittling my suffering.'
- Pause to check if you need to repeat it some more or if any other phrase comes up. If so, continue as before. New phrases may come up quite naturally. Work each through to the end until no new phrases come up and you feel calmer. Try not to stop too early, as this can leave you feeling anxious, irritable or headachy, but do stop if it gets too much for you. If it feels right, you can also use body movements to express how you feel, like wringing your hands or pacing.

It can also help if we allow ourselves to validate our emotions. For example:

- It's completely normal for me to feel so terrified and out of control. I'm not going mad.
- I don't have to keep a lid on my feelings if I don't want to. They're just a normal response to what I'm going through.
- It's okay to keep a lid on my feelings if I need to, but I know my feelings are totally normal.

CHAPTER 5

RELATIONSHIPS AND CANCER

Cancer affects relationships

Relationships are hard to navigate, even without cancer being involved. Layered on top of how difficult they are anyway, cancer's long-term effects can prove fatal to any relationship. Of course, its impact does not have to be so severe, but cancer does seem to change the dynamics of relationships, often enough negatively, but also positively, in some ways and in some cases. Others' experiences confirm this.

To be clear, I mean 'relationships' in the generic sense, to include partners, family including children, friends, work colleagues and, of course, healthcare professionals.

As I start to write, I am aware of a weariness flowing through me as I realise how many times I have pondered on and written about this subject. I am so tempted to use something I have written before here (see, for example, Galgut 2007b, 2007c, 2008, 2010), to save me the emotional pain and the need for self-exposure a worthwhile chapter on this subject actually requires. However, I haven't written much on this topic for a few years, so my views have evolved. An update to self is required. I'll use a few quotes from others, too, some of whom feel differently from me, some of whom feel the same or even more extremely about what cancer's impact on their relationships has been.

'Don't hold back'

I'm aware that the following may not be a comfortable read. It may be considered to be an unusual one, too, especially for someone in my line of work. However, when talking to others before writing this chapter, the consensus was that it needed writing, that I shouldn't hold back, and that some of the issues broached below are taboo and need airing.

Relationships and me – the current position

I suppose I imagined that the impact that cancer was having on my relationships would have lessened by now, 15 years post diagnosis. In fact, not much has got easier, although the hue of things has changed in that I am more resigned to the inevitable – that my ongoing problems, as a result of cancer, will affect my relationships.

To the extent that I am still alive and look 'normal', it is quite often hard for others to accept my ongoing problems unless I am in hospital with a sepsis or looking very ill. Generally, these days, I try to put my best foot forward when I see people, so most can easily avoid the reality of my life, if they so choose. I used to be more honest, but I found that that just caused me problems, so these days I am seldom so with those with whom I socialise. However, I do have friends who know and accept my problems, which I appreciate greatly. It helps that I can meet them from time to time, talk on the phone or FaceTime them. And I have one friend, in particular, who is a lifeline for me.

Almost without exception, however, they have their own problems and their own lives, and we don't live close. The only one who really sees what I suffer on a daily basis is my partner, and she is struggling herself now, as I mentioned in Chapter 4, so obviously, she is not able to support me or understand my predicament in the ways she used to. I pay for support for myself, periodically, but there is a limit to how much of that I can afford.

'I hold grudges'

I would be fooling myself if I didn't admit to myself, at least, that I hold grudges against some people for their historical lack of understanding of what cancer has done to my life, physically, emotionally and financially. I've been told a lot over the years that others coping with cancer's fall-out feel likewise. Typically, people express thoughts and feelings such as, 'she annoys me now. I just can't forgive her', or 'I can't forget what he did, it gets in the way all the time.'

Is this stance psychologically advisable? Well, speaking for myself, probably not, overall. However, I think that sometimes those of us in healthcare expect too much of others and of ourselves, too. We are flawed individuals, all of us. This is a common part of our humanity.

I can and do ask myself why people abandon others when times are hard, and it can help me to think about why and be understanding of their triggers. I remember the people who clearly couldn't cope with my diagnosis and its long-term effects, or those who said repeatedly that I should pull myself together after cancer and that I was exaggerating my problems. Forgiveness is a wonderful thing, if you can manage it, and to some degree I do and have, using strategies such as, 'Remind yourself that they just couldn't cope with your situation, it reminded them of a, b, c or d.' However, I remain angry with some of those people to a greater or lesser extent, whether I want to or not. I'm only human, after all.

Amal, diagnosed with bowel cancer 10 years ago, speaks of her own anger, and why she can't forgive, when she says,

> I get so angry when I think of the people who haven't been able to deal with my cancer diagnosis and the fall-out. Someone who was a friend told me that I had caused the cancer because my diet was bad and I should change it now. There was no sympathy from her, nothing. I told her she was talking crap and after that, I washed my hands of her. I have to see her from time to time, but she is no friend of mine anymore. My mum says I should try and talk to her, but I don't want to and I won't.

'It's liberating'

Interestingly, others have said to me that they find it liberating that I own my anger and my grudges and it helps them feel better about theirs. For example, someone I spoke to not long ago told me that it helped her cope, to repeat frequently to herself how angry it makes her feel when others belittle her suffering. Owning her anger had freed her up to set the bar low with people and to enjoy them for what they had to offer, rather than constantly expecting them to be more understanding.

Holding on to and owning ongoing anger and resentment can also be a useful form of self-protection and, to that extent, personally, I find it useful. What I mean is that if I tell myself such and such a person is not someone I feel positive about, that saves me from having to engage with them and being potentially hurt, undermined or judged, to name just three dangers. If I do have to engage with them, for whatever reason, I remind myself that putting down a boundary is necessary and okay. I will have the necessary contact and not feel guilty if I then remove myself from their company. Sometimes it pays to try to overcome a grudge, and sometimes it just doesn't.

I imagine some of you might be asking, 'Surely, you, the psychologist, would question this stance, wouldn't you?' Well, yes and no, but believe me, I have tried very hard in the past to make relationships work that I would now walk away from. Putting down a boundary and saying, 'This is not good for me and I need to walk away' can also be psychologically liberating. And it has been and is for me, although sometimes very hard. In some ways, cancer has been useful, in that my fuse generally blows more quickly with people than it used to. Before cancer, I would try too hard to make relationships work with people who were no good for me. Now, I generally don't, and I know others who have changed similarly since cancer. And, of course, none of us can really change another person, no matter how much we may want to. All we can do is change ourselves around them, in whatever ways feel right for us.

Reticence about speaking out
When talking to people who have had a diagnosis of cancer, I have found that, at first, some people might say their relationships are unchanged, but after an extended chat and guards being let down, a fair few will complain of lack of understanding and speak of their feelings of resentment and how they feel less tolerant than they did. Some speak of the positives: greater closeness with their partner and the joy of friends or new friends who are very supportive. However, in my experience, those for whom this is their sole experience are in the minority. Of course, positive and negative experiences can exist side by side, and often enough people have told me things such as, ' I'm closer to my partner/child/friend now, but not anyone else.'

More people are affected than we might think

Out of all the people coping long-term with cancer to whom I have spoken over the years, only a handful have asserted that their relationships have not been affected by cancer. Not all feel like me, by any means, but more do than we might think. Samira, diagnosed with breast cancer eight years ago, talking of cancer's long-term psychological effects and others' lack of understanding, says,

> Living with trauma doesn't become easier over time. In fact, it becomes a more isolating experience, as the general assumption is that as time has passed, one should be over it. My diagnosis, operation, chemotherapy and radiotherapy happened eight years ago and whilst I am able to forget for significant periods of time, it doesn't take much to bring back the overwhelming sense of fear and panic, a reaction deemed by everyone, except those I know who have gone through it, to be over-reacting.

Staying silent

I wonder how many others enduring the long-term effects of cancer, with or without sick partners and other problems, are tolerating people in their lives who are unhelpful to them and for them, on all kinds of levels? I also wonder how many of these same people might never speak to anyone about how they really feel. Quite a number, I would think.

A while ago, I spoke to someone in this situation. She disclosed that she had a person in her life she wanted to break loose from because this person was undermining her so much and making her life even more intolerable. However, she was reticent about doing so, in case others judged her. She had never before spoken to anyone about how she really felt about this person, but this relationship was having a hugely negative effect on her. Finding the courage to talk to me about putting down boundaries and getting validation from me about how we all have that right made a huge difference to her confidence levels and empowered her to decide to make some changes. A simple intervention from me, but so powerful for her.

More research evidence is needed on cancer and relationships

There needs to be more reliable research evidence in this area, as well as anecdotal evidence, although there could well be a problem generating reliable data. I have been told often enough by people who have been interviewed that they haven't been honest about their relationships when asked by, for example, healthcare people or researchers for fear of judgement and reticence about whether the person questioning them would understand them or not.

More sensitive, non-judgemental researchers are needed, preferably with insider knowledge of cancer, to help overcome the understandable reticence of long-term survivors of cancer. As John, diagnosed with lung cancer four years ago, said, 'I don't really say how I feel to anyone much, especially to my GP. I don't think he'd get it, judging by the things he says. He hasn't got a bloody clue.'

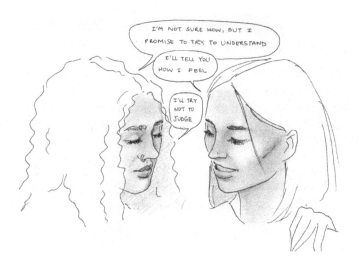

Empathising is key

It's so key that people are able to empathise, or at least attempt to empathise, rather than piling on the platitudes and lack of understanding. You might say, well, as the psychologist, surely you can understand why people can be so lacking in understanding, can't suspend their judgement, etc. I would reply, 'Well, yes, I have explored some of the reasons why, in earlier chapters of this book: fear, lack of experience, entrenched attitudes all abound.'

However, the net result on the recipients of the comments is the same, whether we understand why people are making these comments or not. It's very hard to bear when you are struggling so much. Judgements and recriminations can make us feel very low, depressed and wrong for having the problems we do, even suicidally low.

You don't have to have had cancer to be helpful to someone who has

It's not necessary to have had a diagnosis of cancer to be able to empathise deeply and meaningfully with someone who has and is coping with its long-term effects. It can help hugely if you can admit you can't really understand, but that you'll try your best, rather than trying to pretend you can. That would be an empathic response in itself.

The poem I wrote below, about 10 years ago, echoes many others' thoughts and feelings. I know this because they have told me many times, and used this poem to tell others how they feel.

Please don't...
Please don't tell me how I should feel
Or what I should think about having cancer;
How I should be 'over it' by now;
How I should be more positive;
How I should be grateful that I'm alive.

And please don't say, 'You're over-reacting to your situation.
It's only you who feels like this', or
'It's time you got on with your life.'

How can you know? *You* have never been in my situation.

And please don't ask me what I have contributed to my cancer
Or tell me how brave I've been.
There was no choice is all.
It was just the luck of the draw.

And please don't ask me how my cancer journey has been.
There *was* no journey.
There *is* no journey, because there is *no end in sight.*

And for pity's sake, don't say,
'Well, we're all going to die in the end.
I could get run over by a bus tomorrow.'

It's different

You have never stared death head on.
You have never had cancer.
We are on different sides of the track now.

Tell me instead
That you cannot know what it is like living through this
hell.

Tell me instead that you have an open heart
And an open mind.
That you'll listen,
That you'll try and understand,
Even when what I'm saying sounds preposterous to you.
It is my reality.

And please, please try and look beyond your own fears,
Or if you can't, tell me so.

Having cancer *is* terrifying
And the terror does *not* diminish,
Because the fear that it will come back *is* ever present.

So please, please don't tell me that I'm one of the lucky ones,
That I'll be back to normal soon,

Because my *life* and *I* have been changed forever.

'Your standards are too high'

Well, it's true I have a tendency to expect too much of people –
the flip side of a tendency to expect too much of myself. I'm so
aware of my propensity to expect too much of others that I tend

to go too much in the opposite direction and, for example, not ask for what I need, and tolerate too much.

I am having to ask for support now because there is no choice. A combination of both my partner's problems and my own is far too much. At this point, I need people around me who can make a positive input, but, more importantly than anything else, not judge me at every turn or deny the reality of our situation.

'Solidarity'

Someone very important to me, whom I have known for many decades but not seen for years, came back into my life recently. When I told him about my partner's dementia diagnosis, his response was 'solidarity', among other supportive comments. That's what I need from people I know in relation to my situation.

I know and accept that not many people are able to sustain support and certainly not the hands-on sort. That's hard. I accept people's limitations and their own situations and problems in life. Yes, of course, offering more than kind comments would be wonderful, but it makes such a difference if people are just pleasant, even superficially so, and suspend their judgement as much as possible.

Just one kind comment can bring tears to my eyes, and I know I am not alone in this. Jay, who was diagnosed with lung cancer three years ago, told me recently that a friend of his had come to see him, sat with him, and chatted openly and in a relaxed way, and that had lifted him on that particular day. He said,

> I was feeling so down and unwell and S. came round and asked me how I was feeling and really listened. I know he won't come round again for a while but that doesn't matter. I just felt so understood by him and it made such

a difference. I felt less alone for a moment and it really helped me cope with the day.

Intimacy in relationships and me

There is a distinct limit to what I can cover in this short book, as I mentioned in Chapter 1, and this subject of relationships after cancer and specifically ones in which sex is involved, is a huge topic, no matter how we define what a sexual relationship is or isn't. There do appear to be some common themes, however.

There seems to be a key consensus between those of us who are living with various versions of what I live with that cancer has changed our intimate relationships. By intimate, I don't necessarily mean sexual, and people's views about how important having a sexual relationship is vary. Some are keen to keep a sexual relationship after cancer whereas others are varying degrees of 'not bothered'.

I know significant numbers of people who get fed up that society puts us under such pressure to be sexual, either alone or with others. Suzy, who had bowel cancer eight years ago, is a good example of someone who feels this way. She said, 'I can't stand it when you hear all this hype in the media about sex, almost as if there's something wrong with us if we're not bothered about sex.' Suzy is a post-menopausal woman like me, and it's true that I am nothing like as focused on sex as I used to be. In a way, I find it liberating, one less urge to satisfy. Maybe it is even more liberating for me because I endured so many years of having to have my ovaries switched on and off by adjuvant chemotherapy drugs, post diagnosis. The hormonal fluctuations were unbearable, and my heart goes out to any woman or man enduring these as a result of cancer.

For me, personally, I wouldn't say I'm uninterested in sex or being sexual these days, but if someone were to proclaim that I'd never have a sexual relationship again, I don't think I would be devastated. These days, a combination of constant UTIs (urinary tract infections) and the muscular-skeletal pain that I wrote about in Chapter 4 make any sexual contact hard and often more trouble than it's worth, which is sad, for sure. However, because I am only interested in sexual contact with others as an adjunct to non-sexual intimacy, these days, having lost most of my libido, the act of sex or being sexual has taken a back seat.

Nevertheless, if someone were to pronounce, 'You will never be physically affectionate with anyone ever again', I would find the lack of that possibility very hard. If someone were to say, 'You will never have an intimate relationship with someone ever again', that would be very hard, too. Those versions matter far more to me than sexual contact itself. Had I not had cancer and the long-term problems I have, I don't know how I'd feel about sex. The menopause is a change for most women, and many say sex and being sexual matter less, so who knows. I guess I would probably have had less libido whatever. Again, who knows...

I'm more guarded these days

However, even though intimacy with others, either with or without physical affection, and not involving sex, is important to me, I'm aware that I'm much more guarded with people than before cancer. I've been let down and rejected too many times, so I'd almost rather not risk close relationships for fear I'll be hurt again. And close relationships with people are hard work. Mostly, I'm happier with a cup of tea, a bar of chocolate and a good television programme. Honestly, it's true. And I know I'm not alone. Again, you might say, well, do you, the psychologist, think that's an emotionally healthy way to be? I'd say, to each their own. There's no judgement from me and no right or wrong answer, in my opinion, and I get sick of people telling me there is, in the media and elsewhere.

I'm also aware that I am more comfortable shying away from sexual closeness as my body image is not very good unclothed. It was never robust, but it's worse now because of my scars, radiation damage to my skin and the ageing process on my body. Cancer has definitely had a negative effect on that. It's almost easier to be non-sexual than show any part of my naked body to anyone. So there is definitely conflict in me on this subject, as ever.

However, the other physical problems are more of an issue. Sex could, quite frankly, kill me if I get a nasty, overwhelming UTI after close physical contact with someone, no matter what their gender. I can just imagine the headline, 'Sex gave her sepsis.'

Your issues, Cordelia?

I am aware that there might well be those of you reading this who are tempted to think this chapter is too over the top and must be an exaggeration of how things are for those living beyond cancer diagnoses.

Hopefully, however, the risks I am taking, being open and somewhat unguarded about my own issues, will help others who feel like me, who will recognise themselves in parts or a lot of what I say, and feel validated by my disclosures. As a psychologist, I have certainly found over the years that showing my humanity and fragility with those I support emotionally is often gratefully received, when carefully done. The classic response is, 'If you show your humanity and your frailty, it helps me accept mine.'

I also have the words of all the people who have disclosed the reality of their lives living with or beyond cancer ringing in my ears, especially the ones who have said, 'I daren't say this to my doctor/partner/friend, but I can to you because you have personal experience of cancer.'

'You're running a risk, professionally and personally, so why bother?'

Nevertheless, I can again see a colleague or two, in healthcare or elsewhere, penning a review of this book that misses its point, saying that the author is too unguarded, has too many unresolved issues, sounds too angry and defensive, has too many axes to grind and there is nothing to be gained from her dual perspective. I have also sometimes been criticised for not being objective enough. As I said earlier in this book, I do not believe anyone can be truly objective about anything. It's a concept that holds no water for me. The critic also has an agenda. It may not be mine, but they, too, have an axe to grind, and are far from neutral.

So I expect negative responses but am prepared to take the risk of being very open personally, in order to support my fellow long-term sufferers of cancer. Hopefully, this open stance will also help to enlighten those who are not in the know but are open to knowing more. I'll chunter on in the belief that my approach is more helpful than a dry book in which I take no risks and give nothing away personally. We'll see...

Summary

The following suggestions are by no means exhaustive. Indeed, you may want to add to what follows, based on your own or others' experiences.

It can really help if:

- you can allow yourself to validate how you actually feel about a person or relationship, no matter what anyone else or society tells you you should or shouldn't think and feel
- you allow yourself to speak out as and when you feel the need to

- you allow yourself to express your anger, sadness, etc., if you feel the need to rather than bottling your feelings up because others put you under pressure to do so, or you yourself think it is wrong to do so
- you remind yourself there is no right or wrong way to deal with your strong thoughts or feelings. It is your decision whether you express them or not, nobody else's
- you can set the bar low with people, so you are not constantly disappointed.

It can also help to try an exercise such as the one below.

An exercise that might help communication

The following is an exercise I know many have found useful, including me, at points. It can enable people to say how they really feel without fear of interruption, and can increase the chances that both parties will listen and actually hear what the other is saying. There does, of course, need to be a willingness and openness on both sides to try it. It can be a rewarding experience, but obviously it is not right for everyone.

You can try this with anyone in your personal life. It might help communication between you (even work colleagues, if they agree). You could even try it with your younger children, aged about seven plus, if the strategies are adapted and turned into a kind of game. The strategies take a bit of getting used to, and might feel strange at first, but there is plenty of evidence that exercises such as this one can aid communication between people, and few of us find that easy.

You'll need a stopwatch or something similar.

- Suggest that you and the person in question sit down facing one another somewhere comfortable.
- Tell the other person that you would appreciate them listening to you for two minutes, without interrupting, and then tell them whatever you want to; for example, 'I

hate it when you tell me I should be over cancer by now. I can't be because...' It's better to set an alarm so that they won't clock watch rather than listen to you.

- Invite your partner/family friend/work colleague to say how they feel for two minutes, without you interrupting them.
- When each of you has said your piece, do the same thing again, but this time use your two minutes to sum up what you remember of what the other person has said to you. Even if they feel misunderstood, the person who is listening must not interrupt.
- Take two minutes each again and tell one another what you think of each other's summary. It's very important to do this without judgement. Is it accurate? If it is, say so and thank them for listening and understanding. If it isn't, tell them why it isn't; for example, 'I didn't actually say I'd over-reacted to cancer – I said I've had a strong reaction, and to me that's very different.'
- Take a further two minutes to tell one another what you like your partner/friend/colleague saying to you and what is not okay; for example, 'I really like it when you tell me you understand how I feel. I hate it when you tell me I'm over-reacting.'
- Finally, give one another two minutes to say what each of you has learned about the other from this exercise.

You can adapt this exercise to suit you better. The main thing is to help you and your friends, family, partners and work colleagues, etc., communicate more easily.

Relationships with children during and after cancer

Relationships with dependent children can be very tricky to navigate, at diagnosis and beyond. The responsibility we inevitably feel to protect our children from our cancer, and its effects on us, can easily get in the way of us recognising what our children need from us. It can also be hard, if not impossible, to cope with a distressed child, when we are so challenged ourselves and when those close to us are, too.

Any child with a parent, or any other close adult in their life, who is living with or beyond cancer will more than likely be acutely aware of how cancer has affected the adult. As with all things, children see much more than we might imagine and need as much honesty from us as we can muster, although framed in a form that the child can understand. No one knows a child like the significant adults around them, and they are usually the ones best placed to decide what their child can and cannot understand.

Here is an example of a situation between Rudy and his 12-year-old son, Bumit. He had no idea that the treatments he had for prostate cancer would be affecting him so much, five years on. He didn't say much to Bumit at the time of diagnosis, as he was so young. He assumed he wouldn't notice anything, even the incontinence he suffered badly after the treatments and that he still gets.

A situation arose between father and son recently that started when Bumit started to talk to his dad about the fact that he used to kick a football around with him and that he didn't anymore. Rudy felt guilty because he knew he hadn't really said anything to Bumit about his cancer, and suspected Bumit didn't really understand the problems Rudy had had since all his treatment. However, he also suspected that Bumit had intuited and noticed more than he (Rudy) wanted to admit to himself. So Rudy decided to bite the bullet and talk fairly openly to his son about his physical problems since prostate cancer, including incontinence, in an attempt to explain the lack of football in the garden.

To his amazement, Bumit said he knew all that but he hadn't said anything because his dad hadn't and he didn't want to upset him. Bumit still didn't understand how that meant he couldn't kick a ball around anymore, and Rudy and he had a really open discussion. They ended up hugging and talked about how they could do other things together that they both liked. Interestingly and movingly, Bumit also told his dad for the first time how frightened he had been during his treatment and how he thought his dad was going to die. Rudy apologised to Bumit for not having talked to him more.

Both father and son felt very relieved after that talk, and Rudy determined to be much more open with Bumit than he had been, as he could see it paid great dividends for his child and also for him.

Children who are suffering long-term effects after cancer

While a lot of what I have said in this chapter and this book could be applied to any child coping long-term with cancer and its effects, this is a specialised area, especially when the child is young. There is now growing awareness that children who have been treated for cancer can be affected longer-term by these treatments. No doubt there are also many possible emotional effects, as children grow up and negotiate life after cancer, or indeed, a still present cancer.[1]

---

1   Organisations across the world such as www.macmillan.org.uk, www. cancer.ca and www.cancer.org all have up-to-date information about the long-term effects of cancer on children. In the UK, Teenage Cancer Trust (www. teenagecancertrust.org) specialises in supporting young people with cancer, including after treatment has finished – www.teenagecancertrust.org/about-us/news/young-people-feel-unsupported-after-cancer-treatment

CHAPTER 6

WORK AND CANCER

This topic is not one I can do adequate justice to in this short book. However, it is obviously a hugely important area, since most of us have to work to earn money, and many of us define ourselves, to a greater or lesser extent, in terms of our work. Nevertheless, how cancer's effects, shorter and longer term, affect a person's ability to work as they did before cancer is an ill-considered and little understood subject in the UK and no doubt elsewhere in the world, too. Moreover, the negative psychological consequences of struggling to work, with little or no support and understanding from employers and others, cannot be underestimated.

Challenges in the workplace

There are many challenges for those returning to work after a cancer diagnosis and treatment, no matter what the job. Carrying on working longer term can easily bring with it its own set of problems, too.

Despite the fact that there is legislation in place in the UK to help people go back to work successfully after diagnosis and after or during treatments, it is often not an easy process. Many report experiences shorter and longer term that indicate that the legislation in place is not adhered to strictly, or even at all (Wilson 2018). In essence, both the Equality Act 2010 and the Disability Discrimination Act 1995 provide protection from discrimination. Everyone with cancer is classed as disabled from the point of diagnosis and remains so whether they are pronounced cancer-free or not, so effectively, for the rest of their lives. Additionally, their employer or prospective employer must not treat them less favourably for any reason relating to their cancer. All areas of employment are covered, including recruitment, promotion, training, pay and benefits,

Prior to doing research for this book I had no idea that there was this kind of legislation in existence, and I imagine I am not alone. Interestingly, because it speaks of everyone with cancer being classed as disabled, irrespective of grade or known ongoing presence of cancer, this has encouraging implications for those of us with long-term effects, as well as those coping with the immediate aftermath of cancer. It is, of course, a whole other issue and task getting employers to understand and accept the needs of those coping with cancer's effects shorter and longer term. As Ben Parker, Macmillan Cancer Support's Senior Public Affairs Officer, said to me, 'There is a need to shift the public perception of what living with cancer can mean and to move to improving the understanding that life after treatment can be very different from people's expectations.'

People assume you want to give up work after diagnosis

It is certainly my experience, and that of others I know, that people tend to think that a colossal confrontation with mortality, such as accompanies cancer, will always mean that those of us so affected will want to give up work, run marathons, bungee jump or holiday in far-flung places all the time. Nothing could be further from the truth for many of us, contrary to this conventional wisdom on the subject. On the contrary, large numbers of us want to be as normal as possible. Cancer pulls the complacent 'I'll live for a while yet' rug out from under your feet to such an extent that all many of us want is to get some semblance of normality back as soon as possible, not scale down the side of a cliff face, much as we know that life will never look or be the same again. It is therefore no surprise to me that a Macmillan Cancer Support survey (2016) reported that 85 per cent of its respondents wanted to stay at work after diagnosis. Reasons for wanting and needing to stay in work were: 60 per cent because they wanted to maintain normality and 54 per cent for financial reasons; 45 per cent cited enjoying their job as a reason.

Even when people are dying, it is not uncommon for them to want to continue working for as long as they can, which is a total anathema to many. As Barbara Wilson said in an interview she did for Harley Street Concierge (Working with Cancer 2017):

> Before I had cancer, I remember asking a terminally ill employee why she still wanted to work. And she worked until a fortnight before her death. The simple answer is that it's about feeling normal. Using your brain. Being with colleagues and friends, rather than on your own. There are also financial reasons. But typically – and I can say this based on my own experience – it's about being 'you' again, rather than a cancer patient.

We have a right to work and to be accommodated

This view of a terminally ill employee demonstrates more powerfully than most how those of us who have had or have cancer have a right to work and to be accommodated. However, when special consideration and treatment are needed, the question arises as to what extent these requests are being acceded to. If Macmillan Cancer Support's factsheet entitled, 'Facts and figures: Working through cancer' (Macmillan Cancer Support and YouGov 2010) is anything to go by, there might well be a mismatch between what employers expect and what those of us post cancer or living with cancer can manage: 57 per cent of cancer survivors who were in work when diagnosed had to give up their jobs or change their roles as a result of their diagnosis. This figure was based on an online survey the charity did in 2010 of 1019 people living with cancer, 802 of whom were in employment or education at the time of diagnosis. The two main reasons for needing to give up work or change roles were: not being physically able to work, 43 per cent, and not being emotionally strong enough to work, 25 per cent. Both of these reasons are ones I highlight and explore in other chapters of this book, because they can remain prevalent years after cancer diagnosis and treatment as well as in their immediate aftermath.

What the relationship is between people needing to give up work and lack of understanding of their situation is unclear. However, based on the evidence that is available, common sense would say that there is indeed a link, to a greater or lesser extent. At the very least, lack of understanding can cause low mood and depression, neither of which help any of us cope with a myriad of physical problems caused by cancer's effects. Good communication between, for example, employers, human resources (HR) professionals and employees is key. There are some helpful guidelines that incorporate psychological factors in Barbara Wilson's blog, 'The importance of good communication when supporting an employee with cancer', which is on Macmillan Cancer Support's website.[1]

---

1   See https://community.macmillan.org.uk/blogs/b/the_work_cancer_blog_
    -_advice_for_employers_and_hr_professionals/posts/the-importance-of-
    good-communication-when-supporting-an-employee-with-cancer

'I have struggled increasingly to work'

Although I am self-employed, I myself have struggled to work as I did prior to the bilateral breast cancer I had 15 years ago – and some may say my treatments were much more conservative than many. What has surprised me most is how, having worked a lot for the three or so years after the initial treatments ended, I have struggled increasingly as the years have gone by, due to a worsening of my symptoms because of the longer-term effects of my treatments, described in detail in Chapter 4. I have often wondered how I would have fared if I had been working in institutions, as I did for years, prior to my diagnoses. Badly, I think. Although, the downside of being self-employed has been a big loss of income, over time, due to having to cut down my work and in not having a salary paid monthly, I have not had that pressure of a boss breathing down my neck. As Ben Parker, Senior Public Affairs Officer from Macmillan Cancer Support, said to me, 'Whilst there is often sympathy from employers, there sometimes isn't appreciation that people can continue to face significant physical and emotional challenges after they have finished treatment and returned to the workplace.'

Nor have I had to contend with the judgement of colleagues because they have had to do more work as a result of my struggles to keep things going as before. I do know of teams of workers who have closed ranks to support struggling co-workers, having seen them suffer through the treatment and beyond, which is heart-warming. I also know that even the most patient co-worker can get very fed-up when they are having to pick up the pieces for someone struggling to work post-cancer diagnosis, especially when bosses are unsympathetic and they are under pressure themselves.

Self-esteem and work

I know, from personal experience, as well as from talking to others, that cancer's shorter- and longer-term effects can easily damage self-esteem and self-confidence, across the board, including in the work domain.

I remember that I was desperate to get back to working as I had been prior to cancer, if I could work ethically and well enough (Galgut 2006), and the long-term physical effects hadn't really set in significantly for me at that point. Nevertheless, my self-esteem, on all sorts of levels, had been severely knocked. Somehow, the psychological impact of the diagnosis itself, as well as the damage cancer treatment had done to my body, had wreaked a peculiar kind of havoc with my self-esteem, as had the uncertainty of my future, too. I really needed my work identity to keep me as intact emotionally as I could be. And having to cut down my work as time has gone on, and accept the reality of my situation and eventually give up a large part of my private practice has undoubtedly had a deleterious effect on my self-esteem, although I was 60 when I did so.

'Life had no meaning for me anymore' – Aristos's story

Aristos, who was only 35 when diagnosed with bowel cancer seven years ago, spoke to me of his misery at having had to take so much time off work during and after his treatments, and how much his self-esteem had been ground down by lack of understanding in his workplace.

He was a full-time primary school teacher at the point of diagnosis and loved his job. After the treatments he had, including surgery and chemotherapy, he developed severe gut problems, including faecal incontinence, plus indescribable fatigue. He also had post-traumatic stress, from the awful shock of the diagnosis, etc. When he went back to work, six weeks after the treatments were over, there was absolutely no understanding of his predicament. For example, he couldn't easily take toilet breaks, because people expected him to be back to normal, plus practically, there weren't any available colleagues to watch his class during his absence.

After a month or so of struggling, a decision was made to give Aristos six months paid leave, to aid his recovery. He recognised that he was in no way recovered and that he needed more time, but described that initial phase as,

> ...a nightmare, in that I felt so miserable. Life had no meaning for me any more. Other people were telling me how lucky I was that I had survived, but all I wanted to do was curl up into a little ball and die. It was that bad. If someone had just offered me a tiny carrot, in the form of a few hours a week at school, that would have helped so much, rather than just saying, you can't come into work.

Fortunately Aristos had been given access to some counselling through his GP, who had recognised how shocked and depressed he was, and how desperate. He said,

> I began to understand how a combination of all the changes that had happened as a result of having cancer, including my loss of control over my bodily functions and not being able to work as a teacher at that point, had made a big dent in my self-confidence and feelings of self-worth. I had worked so hard to qualify to be a teacher. It was always my ambition to be one and I was so proud I had made it and cancer had taken all that away. That's how it felt. Counselling also gave me an opportunity to sort my head out about how I could go back to my job. At first, I thought I'd have to give it up, but my counsellor encouraged me not to be so defeatist. That paid off, in that I went back to Occupational Health, knowing I could only realistically work part time,

but with the confidence to ask for what I wanted. It worked out really well in that I was then able to return to work, two days a week and with special considerations in place, because a few of the parents of the children in my class had volunteered to be in the classroom with me, so that I could take toilet breaks. Words can't describe how happy and relieved I was when I found that out.

Returning to work was very scary and hard physically, but Aristos felt so much better, self-esteem-wise for doing so. He said,

Thank goodness I now do teach, only two days a week, but I am so relieved to be able to be back at work. It's all I can manage at the moment, but I feel as though I'm getting my identity back and that's such a relief. Life isn't great. I still suffer a lot from the problems that kept me off work, but they are more manageable now, thanks to the wonderful parents who are with me in the classroom. It turns out that my pupils had really missed me and the parents just wanted me back teaching their kids, but no one had thought to tell me when I was off. Knowing that would have helped so much. Maybe they thought I'd feel pressure to return if I heard that. I don't know. Anyway, now the headteacher and other colleagues at school have to accept my problems. I'm sure it would be easier for them if I was as before, but life is as it is, not least of all for me, and I'm just grateful I can still teach.

Disclosure in the workplace
The problems therein
Such is the stigma around working after and with illness, not just cancer, that I certainly know of people who choose not to disclose they have had cancer to anyone in the workplace,

despite the fact that it can often be excessively hard to keep this private, given the kinds of problems people report after cancer treatment; for example, incontinence, extreme pain or extreme malaise. And, of course, many cope with delayed shock and other psychological effects that can make working as before extra hard.

I certainly understand why people make the choice not to disclose. Having cancer is hard enough without having to cope with people's reactions, including their ignorance about cancer, in addition to coping with the job. I have been told by those who don't disclose that it is just easier for them. Despite the legislation that I referred to earlier, people can also still fear that they will lose their jobs if they reveal their cancer diagnosis. They are often apprehensive that others will judge them differently from before cancer, which is clearly a justifiable worry.

Additionally, in a profession such as mine, in which, as health professionals, we have usually been trained to be 'blank screens' and not disclose anything personal about ourselves, the belief can be that it is wrong to tell patients or clients we have had or have cancer.

The benefits of self-disclosure

However, since cancer, personally I have always offered to disclose my situation to my clients while working as a counselling psychologist. I don't know how I could, practically, have got through working a few weeks after each surgery and each radiotherapy session if I hadn't. For example, during radiotherapy, I had incredibly itchy breasts. I had to disclose what was going on if I were to carry on working, as scratching one's breasts in a consultation with a client is not acceptable, as a general rule! I had to say words to the effect that I was suffering from very itchy skin, and encouragingly, the response from my clients was almost always, 'scratch away'.

I learned a big lesson from my clients then. They said repeatedly that they were sorry I was suffering, but that shows of my humanity made them more able to accept their own frailty, emotional and physical. Additionally, they said they would rather be told the truth about what was going on with me than suspect something was wrong and maybe draw inaccurate conclusions. For example, they might worry that they had done something wrong and that I was cross with them – a common misunderstanding in the face of a blank screen-type of approach from a therapist. No one had ever taught me the benefit of this kind of approach with clients or the risks of a blank screen approach during my years of training, nor had any textbook contained such revelations. In fact, when encouraged to expand on how they felt, my clients often told me that anything less than disclosing my cancer diagnosis and its effects, when relevant, would have been an erosion of the trust that is so vital between therapist and client.

Interestingly, it appeared that I was actually doing a better job of supporting my clients by telling them things about myself and that, carefully handled, my disclosures as a result of cancer were making me a better therapist, albeit a frailer one physically. And these discoveries about what helped and hindered my clients were stimulating and energising at a time when I really needed such input. They also fuelled a desire in me to write about what I was discovering, which, in turn, reignited and reinforced my crusader-writer identity, which drives me to this day.

To this extent, through working, I was reaping one or two positives of cancer amidst all the negatives, not least the many fascinating and often validating reactions I received when I started writing about the psychological impact of cancer from my newly discovered dual perspective. Often, these have been intensely personal, confidential messages, but the reviews of my books in the relevant section of my professional website[2] and my handbook's website[3] give access to many illuminating reviews.

If you don't disclose

Depending on the job, reactions to the disclosure that a colleague has had cancer will differ. However, I have certainly heard it said by the colleagues of those who don't disclose that they know something is up, suspect it's serious, for example, cancer, and that their colleague's behaviour would have been easier to handle if they had been open about what was happening to them.

When you have a job like mine, where the power dynamic is very much in my favour, withholding important information could be considered an abuse of power – it's tricky and unfair if you don't. However, it might also be argued that there are no rights and wrongs here. It's complicated. It depends on the circumstances.

And in essence, it's such a personal and private affair, having cancer. Basically, when it comes down to it, it's just you and the cancer, facing your own mortality, so I would assert that no one has a definitive right to dictate whether someone should disclose their cancer or not. The kind of diagnosis and kind of cancer it is will obviously also inform a person's decision about this.

Rudy's stark situation illustrates that sometimes there is very little choice but to disclose our cancer status, whether we want to or not. He hadn't told anyone at work about his cancer until he was diagnosed with secondary bone cancer.

---

2   www.cordelia.galgut.co.uk

3   www.emotionalsupportthroughbreastcancer.co.uk

He told me,

> I need to say now because I want to keep working. My doctor is telling me I could have years to live and I can take a drug that should slow the spread down, but I know I am going to need time off at points and for the rest of my working life, plus understanding of my symptoms. If I don't tell people at work now, I don't think I can manage.

Personal testimonies

What follows are two more stories of people going back to work after cancer. The first was a teacher and the second a doctor. They serve as further illustrations of some of the problems people encounter when going back to work after cancer, or conversely, having to give up.

....

Sophie, ex-secondary school teacher, diagnosed with ovarian cancer five years ago

At first people were really nice. I just wanted to get back to normal and I was managing fairly well at first. I was only working a few hours a week. I'd missed my pupils and some of my colleagues and just having a normal life. I was totally exhausted from all the chemotherapy and I was struggling with the hormone treatments, but my colleagues were great and with their support, I managed. When the hours I had to work increased from a few hours to a day to a couple of days a week, then three, then the four I used to do, I just couldn't manage. It was too fast and I just hadn't recovered enough as the phasing in period only lasted a month or so. I wasn't ready to go to four days a week by the time I was supposed to be okay.

Nobody really understood why I was struggling so much, including me, but I was having to have loads of time off and I could see my colleagues were getting fed up, carrying the can for me, and I couldn't blame them. I limped on like this for a year or so, but I just hadn't got my energy back as I expected to and had been told I would. I couldn't stand for long without getting exhausted, and I started to get regular dizziness. I got really scared and very worried, because we needed the money and I couldn't imagine life without teaching.

It got to the point that I ended up sobbing in the staffroom, telling colleagues I couldn't cut it anymore and I didn't know what to do. They were really nice then and covered for me such a lot and I'm really grateful to them for that. The headteacher didn't understand and just thought I was work-shy, which caused me a lot of upset and problems. To cut a long story short, I ended up being retired on the basis of ill health, two years after my diagnosis, as my problems had got worse, not better. I'm lucky in that I got a pension, reduced but something. We can't afford to do what we did socially – very few meals out, no holidays, etc., all because I can't teach anymore, due to cancer.

My children are suffering in that they don't get the material things they used to get. I can feel really guilty about that, but the one benefit of this work situation, or lack of it, is that I get to spend lots of quality time with them now. I know how upset and worried they both were about me having cancer and I know they like the fact I'm at home when they get back from school and that matters more than all the stuff they don't get bought these days. Not that they always understand that, though. I'll never be able to have any more children of my own now, due to the treatment I had for the cancer, so my children are even more precious now, if that is possible. I feel so sorry for all the women who lose their fertility as a result of cancer treatment and often can't have their own children. It's so awful and I shudder at the thought that that could have been me.

I do really miss work though. I love being a mum but I want that work identity back. It makes me feel more whole and I really miss it and my self-confidence has taken a big knock now I've lost my job. I've got to find something else to do and ideally make some money, but I've still no idea what, except sometimes I think I could maybe train to be a counsellor and support women who lose their fertility as a result of cancer. I'm not sure I would have the energy to train to do it, but maybe I'll look into that.

It would have been so good if there had been more understanding that life after cancer can be very hard and if someone had warned me this might happen. I'm sure there is some work I can do and I could maybe have stayed in teaching, if there had been more flexible options available. So many people are getting cancer these days. I know other people struggling in their jobs, not saying anything in case they're fired. A friend of mine has been told her performance isn't good enough, recently, so I don't know what will happen to her. It makes me angry. A lot needs to change to help those of us who want and need to work to do so.

....

Elly, doctor, diagnosed with breast cancer two years ago

After my diagnosis, I was determined to get back to work as soon as possible. To be frank, I had had so many patients with breast cancer over the years that I would often think, why not me? It's probably coming my way. And it did. The tumour was small, and the treatment conservative, but harder to deal with than I had realised and I was very tired at the point that I needed to return to work. I stuck to my guns, though, and went back to my busy job as a hospital doctor. I had only told two close colleagues about my diagnosis and in hindsight, I'm not sure that was the best decision, but once I'd made it, I stuck to it. I'd find myself on the ward, almost keeling over with exhaustion and in pain and feeling as though I was slurring my words, with nobody realising why. I felt extremely isolated and quite desperate. That first year was terrible really and one of the close colleagues, who knew about my diagnosis, sat me down one day and gave me a gentle talking to, but she was quite blunt about how I was obviously struggling.

We doctors tend to carry on till we drop. I know it's not a great way to be, but with all the pressures on us currently (in the UK), it's hard not to feel you're letting your patients and colleagues down if you're not trying to be superhuman. I started to accept the toll that expectation of myself was taking on me, after that talk with her. She also persuaded me to get signed off work, to recover properly, which I did. I had a whole month off to sleep, and just try and catch up with myself. I'm acutely aware that I only had surgery, radiotherapy and hormone therapy to contend with and that was bad enough. I certainly hear from others that chemotherapy is extremely gruelling, so I can't imagine what going back to work is like after having that, too.

I felt so much stronger after that month off and at the moment, I'm coping okay. I do get more tired than before breast cancer and I certainly worry about it coming back all the time. I also continue to have pain and certainly don't have the same range of movement as before, which can cause me problems at work. I recently had some counselling and that was a great support and has helped me learn to live with my new state a little more easily.

My advice to anyone wanting to return to work as a doctor after cancer would be to recognise, if you can, that it takes its toll and that it's okay to take some time to recover, in case you mess up on the job and grind yourself into the ground. Even though we are doctors, we're allowed to admit we are human and we suffer like everyone else.

The elephant in the room

How to carry on working, long after treatment has finished, when you are still suffering cancer's effects, or when its effects have worsened, is an issue that is not, as far as I'm aware, one that anybody has adequately addressed, here in the UK. It is the elephant in the room that none of us really talks about. I know people who have just quietly walked away from their jobs, if they could manage financially and, indeed, even if they couldn't, rather than tell employers they couldn't cope anymore.

Short-term strategies, for those affected and their employers, exist, whether they are adhered to or not, but Macmillan Cancer Support's figure of 57 per cent of people who have to give up work or change role seems very telling. It's not clear what percentage of these people changed role within their original workplace, but it would be nice to think that their workplaces had accommodated their colleagues who struggled after cancer diagnosis and treatment. However, the evidence in this chapter alone would seem to indicate to the contrary!

Summary

For those working with or after cancer, the following reminders can be of use, although the list is by no means exhaustive. It can help to:

- allow ourselves to recognise the myriad of problems working with and after cancer can cause us, whether we do so privately or publicly
- recognise that these problems can get worse over time, or just not improve
- remind ourselves that it is not our fault if problems arise in the workplace as a result of non-cancer-friendly systems and structures
- remind ourselves that we have a right to ask for what we need in the workplace, and that there is legislation in place in the UK to support us
- accept that ignorance about living with or after cancer abounds, and that our boss or work colleagues may well not mean to make life harder for us. They just know no better. Their hands may also be tied.

It is our personal decision whether we choose to attempt to raise awareness and/or ask for what we need. There is no right or wrong way forward. It might well depend on factors such as how much energy we have to do so, how risky doing so might be etc.

For those working with colleagues or employees who are living with or beyond cancer it can really help colleagues returning to work soon after cancer diagnosis and treatment, or those living longer term with or beyond cancer, if:

- you can try to suspend your judgement about how your colleague should be performing and try and find out how life is for them, what their problems are, etc.
- you encourage your employees or colleagues to talk openly to you. In order for them to do so, they will need to trust that it is safe to risk this. You may well need to reassure them, especially if you are in a senior position. They may want to talk confidentially and will need to know you will not repeat or record what they have said.

These suggestions are by no means exhaustive, and organisations such as the ones listed in the Resources have lots of information and suggestions that might help you support a colleague suffering shorter or longer term after cancer.

CHAPTER 7

INTERVIEWS WITH A NURSE AND THREE DOCTORS

As part of writing this book, I decided to interview a number of health professionals in order to get their perspectives on the long-term effects of cancer. In this chapter, I focus on four interviews I did with three doctors, two of them surgeons and one a clinical oncologist, as well as a nurse/academic. All four work with cancer patients, either exclusively or have done so for a large part of their professional lives. Because they are all experts in their fields, with laudable and obvious passion for and commitment to what they do, I want their words to stand alone in this chapter with minimum comment from me, unless I think it necessary or can't resist it.

The four interviewees have differing perspectives, depending on each one's particular expertise, experience and personality. However, they also share certain views. Overall, I think they throw an interesting and insightful light on the thorny subject of the long-term effects of cancer and in ways that are highly relevant to this book. I hope you think so too.

The difficulties of speaking out

All three doctors wanted to remain anonymous and not identifiable in any way in this chapter, except to disclose their surgeon or oncologist status. For the purposes of this chapter, therefore, the breast surgeon is called Mr Jones, the gynaecologist, Professor Smith and the clinical oncologist, Dr Evans. Given that I have spoken to a fair number of doctors over the years about cancer-related issues and that most of them haven't wanted to be quoted, even anonymously, not only am I very grateful to the three featured in this chapter for agreeing to be quoted, but it also drives home to me how risky it appears to be to speak out about contentious subjects as a medical person and be identifiable. However, Consultant Nurse, Professor Diana Greenfield, wanted to be identified. I thank her since I am sure not all nurses/academics would have wanted this.

I also spoke to a doctor who has had cancer, for the purposes of this book. Interestingly, the doctor in question was reticent about speaking out from their dual perspective, but did say that they thought there was not enough understanding of cancer's long-term emotional and physical effects within medicine and nursing.

Clearly the four people whose words fill this chapter show a deep and considered understanding of these issues. I am sure they are not alone, but I fear that they may be in the minority.

Long-term effects are real

All four of my interviewees accept that long-term effects exist, both physical and emotional. For example, Mr Jones, the breast surgeon, said, 'We do see long-term effects [with breast cancer], of course. The physical long-term effects to start with and there are also the psychological long-term effects that sometimes change the previous behaviour of a woman or man who's had breast cancer.'

Fear of recurrence

All four interviewees talk about fear of recurrence and how real it is for their patients. Mr Jones talks about the psychological processes that he observes with his patients after diagnosis and treatment for breast cancer, and how the process of realising that it may not be cancer that is causing the pain they are having takes longer to kick in for some people than others. He says, 'For some people, that may happen a couple of years later; for others, five years later; for some it may not happen at all.'

It is interesting that he has identified a transition in some of his patients from thinking that every pain they are feeling is cancer, to starting to consider it may not be. I agree with him that a transition like this is common, as part of learning to live with the fear and the possibility of recurrence and spread.

'A lot more are scared than the ones who verbalise it'

He also replies, in response to my question, 'In what proportion of the women or occasional man you see with breast cancer will you be aware that there are psychological issues, by which I mean fear or terror of recurrence?' 'About a third.' He then asserts, 'With the passage of time, it does get better in all of them, or almost all of them, so if you see the same patient 10 years later, she's not completely hunky dory, but you can see the improvement.' Interestingly, however, Mr Jones and I have an exchange following on from his assertion that women improve over time, in relation to coping with fear of recurrence, which shows that he knows this whole issue of fear of recurrence is not black and white.

Continuing on from Mr Jones saying he observes that a third of his patients have emotional issues, the conversation continues,

Me: 'It's interesting, because I think some people are embarrassed to admit fear beyond a certain point.'

Mr Jones: 'Maybe, but you do see that their attitude has changed.'

Me: 'Inevitably, as time passes, you get more used to it, it's like the death of someone.'

Mr Jones: 'Correct.'

Me: 'It's like you learn to live with it.'

Mr Jones: 'With the passage of time you become better.'

Me: 'You live alongside it better.'

Mr Jones: 'Correct.'

Me: 'You may be as frightened of it.'

Mr Jones: 'You just don't express it so much. It doesn't come to the forefront [as much].'

He also said, at another point in my interview with him, that 'a lot are scared and more than the ones who verbalise it. I'm pretty sure of that'. So he is clearly aware of how complex fear of recurrence is psychologically, and reflects on the subject.

'There's a fear of recurrence in the patient's mind'

Mr Jones also gives me an example of what might happen with a patient in a consultation. He says,

> Well, this is the kind of thing somebody could say during the consultation. A patient might say, after five years on Tamoxifen, and at the point of stopping it, 'Are you sure I don't need it for longer?' So she's been thinking about it. She's still realising that there's a chance of recurrence. There's a fear of recurrence in the patient's mind. Perhaps more than there should be. I don't know what it should or shouldn't be, but clearly there's something there.

Mr Jones also identifies another very real issue for those of us who have had breast cancer (and other cancers). He says,

'I think it is difficult for them to know whether what they are feeling is real or imagined.'

What he says is totally right, as I well know. I need to be aware that a symptom I have could be more cancer. It probably isn't, but if it's a lump, clearly it needs checking. If it is more generalised pain, it can be impossible for me to rationalise it, because there is always that tiny element of risk in doing so. Sometimes I can and mostly do ignore those symptoms, but I'm always aware that the only way to be reassured is to see my breast surgeon. And, of course, Mr Jones is aware of this. He says, 'Until they get the person [surgeon] to examine them and assess a combination of their ultrasound, blood tests, what have you, and [I] tell them, I can feel there's something there, but you know it's not due to recurrence. Only then can the patient be reassured.'

'Cancer, can you think of anything worse?'

Professor Smith is a gynaecologist who sees a significant number of cancer patients. His attitude to fear of recurrence is very clear. 'Cancer, can you think of anything worse? This aspect of it doesn't just stop. It's constantly there, in the background, and then there's this constant reminder of it, every time you see anything related to that disorder.'

'They're petrified it's going to come back'

He is also aware that the long-term emotional effects of cancer are going to become more and more of a problem, as people survive longer. He continues,

> In a way, suffering after cancer is becoming a more prevalent issue. We're now having more people where cancer is being treated and it can be that they may be defined as cured, but there will be physical cure and then the other problem

will be whether they are psychologically cured, because I've certainly seen a number of patients where they've been told their cancer has gone, but quite obviously, from their behaviour, they're petrified it's going to come back, and that is not being addressed because they're being told, 'Well, it's physically gone'.

'It is a very rational fear'

Professor Smith also recognises that, 'If they come and say I'm still worried about this, well they're told that's not a rational fear, but of course it is a very rational fear, because this is something they lived through; it is a possibility and then how do they get help?'

He continues,

The other group, which is a real issue, is where the cancer exists, they're being treated, they're on long-term treatment, oral let's say, and we see this with metastatic breast cancer. They're told by the oncologist, this could be 10 years, it could be 20 years, it may not even get worse, but it's there and that's a very scary thing, because it's present. Somebody has said there is a clock ticking and at some stage, the treatment may not work and they have to live with that; and again, the lack of support for that group creates stress and I think the key issue is how can these patients be supported when really it's perceived that the treatment has worked, so why is there a problem?

Resistance to accepting long-term effects

Professor Smith also broaches the subject of resistance within medicine and the healthcare community at large to accepting the existence and impact of long-term effects and why this is, and touches on areas I addressed in Chapter 2. He says,

My suspicion is that we like to deal with tangible things, also personally, we doctors would like to be able to do something... It's probably that the caregiver feels powerless to do anything. Often, if you feel powerless about something, you don't want to confront it. It's much easier just to deny it exists, because, in a way, it's your own vulnerabilities [at stake].

Also, he asserts, 'The caregiver may not understand what's going on or what concerns the person has or what support they need.' When I ask, 'What might help a medic in that situation?' Professor Smith's reply is,

First of all, you've got an issue in terms of acknowledging it exists. That's primary. That's the biggest issue by far and it's something that concerns a substantial number of patients, because I would argue that a doctor who knows those concerns exist for the patient would want to do something about them. Again, it's that idea of doing something. And the second thing is having the tools to deal with it.

In response to me saying it's a tall order to support psychologically as well as medically, Professor Smith says, 'All the doctor can do is to direct to the right person or right GP.'

And, in relation to lack of support for people suffering the long-term psychological effects of cancer, for example, fear of recurrence, he says,

It's knowing where people can get support. That's a great deficiency. A huge issue. It's going to become a bigger and bigger issue. We're going to get more and more cures, more and more stable cancers. I don't think we've even got a name for it. I don't think we've quite got our heads round it. That's where cancer is going.

'Being disease-free is not the same as being free of the disease'

Professor Diana Greenfield talks about 'the lack of parity of esteem' between the medical and psychological as in, 'we've got a big gap in services between what's provided medically and what's provided in terms of psychological support'. She continues, 'Patients' psychological and emotional needs are rarely given the same priority, despite high levels of distress experienced by cancer patients, and this can be demonstrated through the poor availability of clinical services to meet these needs.'

She then adds,

Some patients with really marked distress or mood problems are likely to experience a delayed recovery, with implications for a postponed return to work or other meaningful activity and with implications for their physical health and recovery. We know that a significant proportion is consuming health resources (such as repeated visits to their GP) because their emotional and psychological needs, associated with having cancer or having had cancer, are not being met.

Furthermore, she continues,

The incidence of cancer is increasing year on year and we are currently not meeting today's need, let alone planning for tomorrow's. It's a concern. It's imperative we reconsider how we manage the continuing growing cohort of people with cancer treatment-induced late effects – including the emotional and psychosocial effects. If there's one thing healthcare professionals should remember when caring for a patient affected by cancer, being disease-free is not the same as being free of the disease.

Their role in relation to the emotional long-term effects of cancer

'I feel it is my responsibility to ensure that at some point, they normalise more'

Mr Jones does think it is part of his job as a surgeon to manage his patients' ongoing fears. He is acutely aware that 'All patients are anxious after a diagnosis. They all fear that it could be a symptom of local recurrence or metastatic breast cancer [spread to organs, bones, etc.].' As a result, he says,

> I feel it is my responsibility to ensure that at some point, they normalise more, they appreciate that, fine, if you get a new symptom, it needs to be checked, it's true, but you must realise at some point that, yes, you are going to be developing symptoms that are due to other things than cancer. Just because you had cancer before doesn't mean that everything you feel in your body is due to cancer.

He does acknowledge, however, that, 'I don't think there is a lot I can say to make them believe that.'

Mr Jones clearly does want to offer some emotional support, and I think he is probably unusual in this, as a surgeon. He has also reflected over time on how he acts with his patients in relation to, for example, fear of recurrence and spread. He sees it as his role to pick up on anxiety he detects in his patients. For example, he says,

> There are a lot of people who ask questions; not directly, but [they'll say] 'it's three years now, is there a chance it'll recur?' That shows they do think about it. That means to me that they are anxious about it. They're anxious about the possibility of it coming back. That would be a prompt for me to probe it a little bit further, perhaps, to find out exactly how anxious they are. Is it something that occupies their

mind all the time or is it something they think about just before they come to my appointment?

This comment prompted a jokey exchange between us, me suggesting he was a bit of a psychologist, to which his reply was, 'I don't think I am.' However, he did disclose that,

> Yes, I've got better at it over the years. Let's face it, 20 years ago, I probably wasn't as good at it, but you do see a lot of people and you see the ones where actually it's in the back of their minds 24 hours a day, and there are others who think about it just before they have an appointment to see you, and I think you get better with experience, at knowing who is feeling what.

'Otherwise, I would be a breast operator, not a doctor or a surgeon'

Overall, in relation to long-term effects, be they emotional or psychological, Mr Jones says,

> I'm not in the business of ignoring them because 99 per cent are going to be fine; it's very important to deal with the 1 per cent. No, you do need to figure, who is the one who has a recurrence? In the other patients, the symptoms are because of the treatments, but in that patient, they do have a recurrence. And you've got to be clever enough to figure that out.

He admits it's a lot of pressure and very hard, but ends with, 'I do accept that it's part of the job. Otherwise, I would be a breast operator, not a doctor or a surgeon.'

'You have to initiate'

Professor Smith, the gynaecologist, definitely sees it as his role to broach taboo subjects with his patients who have had cancer; for example, those related to the long-term effects they suffer, either emotional or physical. And, of course, the two are inseparably intertwined. He says,

> You have to initiate and ask someone if they have specific problems in those taboo areas: do you have difficulty with passing urine frequently, or about the vagina, is it dry, is it sore? If someone like me doesn't initiate asking about those areas of the body, the patient may well feel too embarrassed to.

He continues,

> Unfortunately, patients are started on things like Citalopram for anxiety, a lot of patients are on that. There's a lot of polypharmacy and drug therapy and it's primarily because it's not accepted that the symptoms they are complaining of are very reasonable. I don't think there is even an acknowledgement that it is very reasonable. I can't think of anything more scary [than the fear of getting more cancer].

'It's easy to focus on all the new patients'

Dr Evans, the clinical oncologist I interviewed, who is aware and concerned, comments that, 'You know, I think oncologists, many of us just don't appreciate that what we do to patients has incredible effects on their physical and mental wellbeing. It takes such a long time to recover, or sometimes it doesn't'. He then goes on to pinpoint one of the reasons for this when he says, 'It's easy to focus on all the new patients that are coming through your clinic every day and not consider the ones you've already treated. It's stopping one day, when your patient comes back and saying, 6, 12, 18 months after they've finished treatment, how do you feel?' He is also aware that, 'When my breast cancer patients come back and see me annually after a mammogram, the psychological effects of the build-up to it can be awful.'

The long-term physical effects
All four of my interviewees spoke about the kind of physical long-term effects they encounter in their patients after cancer treatment.

'We see changes in the body after someone is treated for breast cancer'
Professor Smith highlights something he sees. He said,

> Yes, there is something which happens, and this is long-term. I've only seen it in breast cancer and something happens to the way their body responds. Now I don't know whether it's that, or [there is] some strange inflammatory thing which has started. I don't know what causes it, but certainly we see changes in the body after someone is treated for breast cancer, and completely separate from the breast cancer itself. It seems to stem from that point [the treatment].

He continues,

> I thought there was a name for one syndrome, it's one of these unknowns, we don't know what the cause is and it's associated with breast cancer and I've heard that from a professor of oncology who mentioned it and said this thing exists. There's no known treatment for it.

He then goes on to highlight why acceptance of the syndrome is difficult within medicine,

> I think that what has to be acknowledged is that at the root of what's important about this is that, unfortunately, in

medicine, or science in general, we like to define a problem, know how many people are suffering from it and only then, with that basis, can awareness occur.

'The longer they survive, they have to put up with these side effects'

Mr Jones, the surgeon, also sees the long-term physical effects in his patients, along with fear of recurrence. As well as speaking about changing emotional effects over time, he talks about the physical effects of longer-term survival:

> The longer they survive, they have to put up with these side effects or adverse effects of treatments. And also, the treatments, or some of the treatments we try, they take longer to complete, so people have to face the adverse effects of treatments for much longer. Hormone therapy, for instance, 10 to 15 years ago, it was a five-year course, now it's 10 years. I think the chances are it will increase in length in future.

Mr Jones goes on to dispel the idea that only people with recurrences have long-term effects, reiterating that,

> The normal treatments that we have today for breast cancer, like surgery, radiotherapy, hormone therapy, chemotherapy, they do cause a lot of long-term symptoms. I tell you, when I was first trained, the going theory was that up to a third of women having breast-conserving surgery may report pain afterwards, whereas, I mean, I think that's wrong. All of them do.

He then validates changes in symptoms over time when he says,

> And things change and then, of course, the sensitive patient is going to say, 'This change is maybe a recurrence and it's a rational symptom, or a rational interpretation of

a symptom, why should it change five years later?' But it does, it does.

Getting consent

Dr Evans, a clinical oncologist specialising in breast and lung cancer, speaks a lot about the long-term effects he encounters and also about the difficulty of having to decide which treatments to use, given their ability to cause long-term effects, some more serious than others, including even death. He starts by describing cancer treatment consent forms. He says, 'The consent forms we use for treatments are mindful of the side effects of those treatments, whether it's chemotherapy in leukaemia or radiotherapy in breast cancer.' He elaborates, 'When a patient consents to treatment, it's ensuring they have the understanding and the information to be able to make that informed decision to proceed.' He then details some of those effects: 'It [for example, adjuvant breast cancer chemotherapy] can affect their fertility, through early menopause. It can increase the risk of cardiovascular disease, their risk of a second cancer, and the risk of life-threatening infections. All those things are typically listed on the consent forms we use.'

Radiation itself causes genetic mutation

He then goes on to talk about the early and late effects of radiation treatment and how these are defined. He says,

> As a clinical oncologist, I specialise in all the non-surgical aspects of cancer care including radiotherapy. My radiation training included education on the early and late effects of radiotherapy on the human body. Acute radiation side effects are typically defined as side effects lasting up to 90 days post radiotherapy and commonly include skin reaction, fatigue, tiredness. Late side effects,

on the other hand, are the ones which gradually develop as time ticks by and the years (hopefully) roll on since the patient completed their treatment. These are normally secondary to the radiotherapy's effects on normal tissues which include tissue hardening and fibrosis formation within the irradiated tissues. This can have a significant effect, for instance, in patients who have had their breast irradiated. Over the course of years, their breast can become harder, the tissues less elastic, the breast itself can shrink compared with the untreated side, pigmentation changes can develop in the skin and, consequently, significant cosmetic changes occur. What also becomes clear when you monitor a population of patients who have had radiotherapy is that other serious conditions seem to occur more frequently in that population. For example, the incidence of cardiovascular disease increases compared with that of a matched non-irradiated population.

He continues,

And also we must remember that radiation itself causes genetic mutation. When we deliver radiotherapy at a curative dose to treat cancers, we also inevitably irradiate surrounding normal cells. It is rare, but these normal cells can mutate and over the course of time, typically after 10, 20 years or more, can go on to become cancers themselves. We don't tend to see this effect within the high dose radiotherapy field, but as you move away from the edge of your field into the surrounding normal tissues, it's these which have received a lower dose of radiation, and it's within these tissues that it seems to occur more often. It's this effect which leads to the late toxicity we term radiation-induced second malignancies.

When I asked Dr Evans what kind of second malignancies he sees, he said, 'Lung cancers, cancer of the oesophagus, breast cancers and even radiation-induced sarcomas.'

'Radiotherapy scatter in terms of radiation, absolutely'

Generally, 'scatter' of radiation to other areas of the body, other than the one that is being treated, is a 'no go area' when I have raised it with medical people. However, Dr Evans is clear when he says,

> Scatter in terms of radiation, absolutely. If you put dose-recording devices on patients receiving radiotherapy, you'll detect scatter, and this can include on their head, even when you're irradiating their abdomen. You do get dose at other areas and we are becoming more mindful of this whilst delivering radiotherapy. We have become more advanced, and now utilise what is termed image-guided radiotherapy where we now use more X-ray-based images during treatment to help localise the target. We now use cone beam CTs to help target cancers more accurately, and this does involve patients having more scans and therefore larger doses of radiation.

However, he continues,

> But you have to put it into context and it depends on the context you use. If you put it into the context that they're receiving a radical dose of radiotherapy to cure them of cancer, or at least reduce the risk of their cancer returning, then the dose that you're delivering for that kind of makes the dose you're using to take pictures seem considerably smaller and less significant. So, it's different scales of magnitude, but you still have to be able to justify it. As a clinician you have to be incredibly conscious of the dose

you're using with your patients. You have to be able to justify it, which means you have to feel it's worthwhile for their treatment and the overall benefit they'll get from having their treatment more accurately. What needs to be considered is that in some centres, in some countries, there's probably different levels of consideration of that fact.

'Default [settings] can be considerably higher and potentially more difficult to justify'

Dr Evans continues,

What's also interesting is that the machines themselves, when they're delivered from the manufacturer, the standard settings that they have for taking, for instance, cone beam CTs, from our experience, when we've looked at the those default settings compared with those we've created ourselves, is that the doses delivered using the default ones can be considerably higher and potentially more difficult to justify. If you therefore don't review these settings within your institution, you may be delivering unnecessarily high doses of radiation in the context of your own, on treatment, cone beam CT imaging.

It's a hard situation for Dr Evans to accept, in that, as he says, and I'm sure he's not alone:

The whole principle of medicine is that you do no harm and you have to be able to justify the clinical decisions you make in treating your patients. As a cancer doctor, when I'm with a patient discussing the merits of chemotherapy, radiotherapy or immunotherapy, if I can't justify why I want to do X, Y or Z, then I really shouldn't be thinking about doing it.

Late cardiac effects of radiation for lung and breast cancers

When I raised with Dr Evans whether there was anything to do with the late physical effects of cancer treatment that we didn't know last year but has since emerged, his response was,

> Yes, what's currently emerging in lung cancer is the late effects radiotherapy can have on the heart following curative radiation treatment for lung cancers. What's becoming evident is that our eye, if you like, is focused on the ball in terms of eradicating the cancer. Whilst we are meeting what we currently consider the safe dose constraints of the normal lung and heart tissues, when you look at the long-term outcome data, some patients who survive their lung cancers then go on to die from cardiovascular disease, which might have been exacerbated by the radiation dose they received to their heart. So, it's now become an area of keen interest as to ways in which we can minimise cardiac toxicity in the context of lung cancer radiotherapy treatment. As cancer treatment has evolved, the focus has always been on curing the cancer, making patients free of their cancer so they can get on with living their lives. What we're being more conscious of now, I think, through the success of curing cancer, is that patients can then die of a complication which could be linked, and sometimes is, to the radiotherapy treatment they've received.

He continues by explaining,

> Within the scientific literature, there are no better examples than the late cardiac effects of radiotherapy for early breast and lung cancers. But you don't want to throw the baby out with the bathwater and begin to restrict the dose that you deliver to the cancer to avoid radiation dose to the heart. If you do, you will reduce the chance of curing the cancer,

and then patients will die of the disease which might have been cured. You therefore have to achieve the right balance, where you're maintaining the radiation dose to the cancer so as to maintain your chance of cure, whilst delivering as low a dose as possible to the normal, healthy tissues around the cancer so as to minimise late toxicities.

'It's only through the success of cure that you become conscious of the sequelae of achieving that cure'

When I sympathised with Dr Evans about what a difficult area this is, constantly trying to achieve the right balance and do as little damage as possible, while attempting to cure or manage the cancer, his response was, somewhat poignantly, 'Yep, but again, you know, it's only through the success of cure that you become conscious of the sequelae [consequences] of achieving that cure.'

Dr Evans also reflects on the fact that he is a relatively young oncologist,

> ...but there are oncologists who are just retiring now, at the end of their career after 30 or 35 years and it's the late effects of their treatments that we're now conscious of, so it's adapting what they've done to achieve these cures, and in doing so, reducing the risks of the late side effects we might see later.

What's the right length of treatment?

Like Mr Jones, Dr Evans also mentions the fact that drug treatments are going on for longer and longer, for example, Tamoxifen for breast cancer, and raises the contentious but important issue of the role of drug companies in relation to this. He says,

I can understand pharmaceutical companies want their drug to be given as maintenance for as long as possible. However, scientific sort[s] of clinicians want to be able to scientifically justify or at least question what's the right length of treatment, but it conflicts with their [the drug companies] interest, yes?'

It's 'we', not 'them' and 'us'

Professor Diana Greenfield, Consultant Nurse, is aware and concerned about how our approach to those suffering long-term can be negatively affected by some entrenched attitudes still too commonly present in healthcare (highlighted in Chapter 2). For example, she stresses the need 'not to be complacent enough to think it's "us" and "them"'. She reinforces this by saying, 'The first thing a professional should recognise is that it's "we", not "them" and "us".' She also believes that it's important to explain that, 'I haven't had cancer (yet)' and that 'you're not an expert till you've been through it.'

Professor Greenfield is also very aware of the statistics regarding cancer: 'The statistics are 50/50, one in two of us will now get cancer in our lifetime.' She is therefore aware of the risks for herself and her family, and this fact informs how she thinks and feels about supporting those coping with cancer's effects longer term, which she does, in her clinical role. She says,

It shouldn't be difficult, as healthcare professionals, to show empathy: just put yourself in their shoes. A patient, a young woman, who was treated for an ovarian germ cell tumour two years ago, reported to me in clinic the other day something her GP apparently said to her: 'It's time you got over it now.' If it's true, then this is pretty unforgivable and demonstrates a number of training needs, compassion being the first.

'We've got increased survival [rates]'

Regarding the long-term and late effects of cancer, she says,

> Thanks to modern medicine and advanced science, there are very many people living well beyond cancer. But there are other people living beyond cancer who may not be well, often due to the consequences of treatment. This is a silent and growing epidemic and current health services are not well equipped to deal with people affected by cancer.

She says,

> The statistics speak for themselves. We've got increased survival [rates]; many cancer types which have improved survival rates as a result of better medical management, such as screening, early detection, improved treatments, monitoring, supportive care and multi-disciplinary team working. However, long-term and late effects of treatment have meant there are numbers of people living with physical and psychosocial problems and care systems have not developed in response to dealing with these problems.

She continues, 'Managing cancer treatment consequences is now a priority in the latest cancer strategy in England, with similar programmes in all four home nations. This is positive, but progress is slow.' The reason she gives for the lack of progress is,

> It takes a long time to operationalise a complete change in culture and this is particularly challenging because of the competing challenges and priorities in a time of austerity. One main solution is to shift the responsibility of dealing with late effects to primary care, but resources, drivers and incentives have not yet followed, let alone training and workforce initiatives on the back of other pressing initiatives in primary care.

Who's responsible?

She also highlights an issue regarding which healthcare professionals are responsible for caring for people at risk or who have complex treatment consequences. She says,

> This is a significant concern. Currently the main solution is to transfer responsibility to primary care services. This may work for relatively straightforward patients, but I think it is unrealistic to expect GPs to have expert knowledge about late effects and managing patients with multiple complex needs, all of which may require specialist input. From the outset, the specialist oncology team are currently not effectively or routinely communicating late effect risks with their patients or their GPs. That's mainly because many oncologists are focused on the primary disease and its management. Plus they don't often see their patients long enough to observe or understand significant late effects and the impact these have on an individual's health and functioning.

She continues, in support of oncologists,

> With some of the new cancer care pathways, patients may be discharged sooner or transferred to GPs for shared care, and oncologists may not see the issues. So it's not necessarily that they're not taking responsibility because they don't want to; they simply aren't fully aware of the late effects associated with the treatments they are giving.

However, she also points out,

> Additionally, many cancer doctors don't see screening and managing for late effects as their responsibility, and GPs aren't being given the clinical information or the resources to do it either, so there's a problem. There is currently very little, if anything, in oncology doctors' training, or in GP

training, on cancer treatment late effects, and that is not in the best interest of our cancer patients.

Absence of the disease is not the same as being well

Professor Greenfield highlights, in the quote above, that being cancer-free doesn't necessarily mean experiencing a good quality of life. Leading on from this, she says, 'Normalising the experience, giving permission, for example, to say, "It's okay to feel rubbish", can be reassuring. Having an honest and meaningful conversation about expectations for recovery [physical and emotional] can also be really helpful', especially if it is, 'built into the routine cancer pathway [appointments], and given as much parity as, for example, follow-up scans.'

My thoughts...

Although, as I said at the start of this chapter, I want these doctors and this nurse's words to stand alone, without too much analysis and interpretation from me, I do wonder how much the kinds of things they have said in their interviews represent the views of those who dare not speak out in healthcare, even anonymously. It's hard for me to say, but judging by the conversations I have had over the years with others in medicine and nursing about these issues, they are not alone. I also know that there are those who are speaking out and trying to effect change, often in the face of opposition. While I did not interview a mental health professional for this chapter, thinking that my psychologist voice throughout the book was quite enough, I do know that others in mental health also echo the kinds of views expressed by the voices here.

The elephant in the room is the fear of speaking out and being identified, and of speaking out, even anonymously. I think that this fear and why it exists is very complex. One possible explanation might be fear of a fiercely dominant culture in healthcare – the one I focused on in Chapter 2 – that does not tolerate challenge, that fails to realise how potentially damaging its attitudes are, and that punishes those who do speak out in a variety of ways. There is also a huge rank-closing culture in healthcare, which might explain some of the reticence. I'm just not sure.

And yet, the kinds of issues the doctors and nurse in this chapter raise and explore are vital ones for us all to engage with openly if anything is ever going to change for the better in relation to the long-term effects of cancer. So where do we go from here? More people daring to speak out as much as possible, I guess. How optimistic am I that this will ever happen? Well, that is a whole other question...

Summary

For those suffering the long-term effects of cancer, the following are tips for talking to doctors and nurses. Remind yourself:

- Most doctors and nurses will want to help, but they may well not know how to.
- They may need educating by those of us with long-term effects, but it's reasonable to expect them to listen and to try to help.
- There will be a limit to what they can do, but it is totally reasonable to ask:
  - For acknowledgement of what you are suffering, for example, 'It would help me to know that you accept that long-term effects exist' or 'It would help me to know that you believe my symptoms are/might be related to the long-term effects of cancer.'

    – For a referral to their colleagues who can help with specific symptoms, be they emotional or physical. You could say any of the following, for example:

'Since my cancer diagnosis and treatments, I have continued to suffer from (extreme) pain that prevents me doing lots of things and I can easily feel depressed because my life is so limited these days.'

'These symptoms have got worse over time, not better.'

'Are you able to offer me some help with these problems, please?'

'I understand that you may not be able to help/support me yourself, but please could you refer me on to a colleague of yours who might be able to help?'

If you find your doctor or nurse is not being as understanding and supportive as you might like, you could,

- Try to speak to or email the person/people/practice manager or equivalent in the hospital/GPs surgery concerned, and lay out your concerns. You have a total right to do this and to be taken seriously.
- Contact the helpline of a charity such as Macmillan Cancer Support[1] to talk through your concerns and to get advice (see also the Resources at the end of this book).

For healthcare professionals:

- It is often very useful if you are able to acknowledge the reality of cancer's long-term effects with your patients. In many cases this, in itself, will be helpful to them.
- Try not to give yourself a hard time if there is no more you can do.

---

1   www.macmillan.org.uk

- Try not to worry about admitting you don't know. People with long-term effects might well value that honesty and find it validating of their situation. The least supportive healthcare professionals are often deemed to be those who assert things with great confidence when they are actually ill-informed and unsure. Most patients will see through this anyway, so I am told.
- Charities such as Macmillan Cancer Support can be a great help to those of us in healthcare as well as to patients.

CHAPTER 8

IF ONLY: THE EXPERIENCE AFTER TREATMENT FOR MALE CANCERS

Simon Crompton

Health journalist Simon Crompton here examines the male experience of living with the effects of cancer treatments.

Would I have become a health journalist if my dad hadn't died of prostate cancer? Probably not. Like many of those who work in healthcare and its orbit, my career course was partly determined by the health experiences of those close to me.

Of course, it isn't just the dying bit that has such a strong impact on the family and close friends of those who have cancer. It's the living bit. It's that day-to-day experience of living with a disease and its aftermath that relatives view at close hand – never sharing the unique viewpoint of the person with cancer, never exactly understanding how it feels, but knowing that it achingly matters, and knowing that this is the bit that doctors never talk about.

And if, back in 1983, it was the dying bit that affected my family most, when we lost Dad at the age of just 62, today it's the living bit I think about more. I think about those five years between his diagnosis and death, and all those little clues to what he was going through and how he was feeling that I subconsciously picked up on but chose to ignore because I was 18 and life had to go on. I think of it more since my sister was diagnosed with breast cancer 10 years ago, and then with another breast cancer one year ago – and see again the challenges of life continuing with the background noise of cancer and its treatments droning away, sometimes blaring.

The way the world looks changes

It's always been clear to me that living with and after cancer changes not just your life but also the way the world looks and feels. It's true of any major illness. As I write this, I have just spoken to a man with multiple sclerosis for whom life is now simply not worth living as a result of erectile dysfunction – a symptom of his condition. It's not just that he can no longer have sex with his girlfriend. He's lost his sense of identity. The things that gave him a sense of self revolved around a perception of masculinity and now, because of his disease, that idea of himself is impossible to live up to.

Those circumstances may be specifically male. Some may find the thought process difficult to empathise with. But it is true, and by no means unique. A world-warping shift can be sparked by all types of illness, for both genders, and can continue eroding sense of self and quality of life for many years after people are supposed to be 'better' or 'back to normal'. Your health affects who you feel you are and your place in the scheme of things.

This has always been an area neglected by researchers, and too often forgotten by health professionals. Addressing problems beyond the physical cure, or the palliation of symptoms, requires a personal involvement and a willingness to tackle complexity that health services are poorly designed to address.

Maybe the fact that so many people with cancer struggle after treatment – and sometimes feel guilty that they don't feel grateful for simply being alive – is more shocking to us than for other diseases because so much money and attention is focused on the cancer cure, and so little on what happens to people afterwards. We really don't know what the experience is for the vast majority of people after cancer treatment. Only in the past 20 years have trials of cancer treatments started to systematically evaluate their effect on long-term quality of life, as well as survival. Recent analysis in the *American Economic Review* (Budish, Roin and Williams 2015) concluded that pharmaceutical company investment is still distorted away from studying the long-term effects of treatments.

What research tells us about the long term

We do have some general indications that things are far from easy. Around half of those with cancer live for at least 10 years after diagnosis, but at least one in four have poor health over the long term. People with cancer are 60 per cent more likely to attend Accident and Emergency than the general population (Chitnis *et al.* 2014).

Beyond those broad strokes, there is some evidence about the long-term effects of some treatments – pain, incontinence, infertility and impotence, heart problems, depression – which people live with for the rest of their lives. A 2016 study in the *Journal of Clinical Oncology*, for example, showed that people with multiple myeloma, non-Hodgkin lymphoma and cancers of the breast, kidney, lung/bronchus and ovary are up to 70 per cent more likely to develop cardiovascular disease as a result of their treatment than someone who has not been diagnosed with cancer (Armenian *et al.* 2016).

It goes without saying that, on diagnosis, cure should be the first item on the agenda for both patients and health professionals. The problem is that discussion rarely goes beyond this in hospitals. Because knowledge about long-term effects of treatments is scanty, and because cancer specialists have an interest in promoting what they are good at rather than options that make decisions complicated, treatment choices are often made quickly.

The experience of men with genitourinary cancer

I have spoken to many people who have been treated for cancer who now wonder whether, if they had known enough about the consequences of treatment, they might have chosen a different course. The feeling is common across all cancers, but I have encountered it particularly among men affected by cancers of the genitourinary system. Long-term effects such as urinary and bowel incontinence and sexual problems often follow radiotherapy and surgery for prostate cancer. A 2017 study in *Cancer Medicine* found that they commonly continue 10 or more years after treatment (Jang *et al.* 2017).

If only they'd had more chance to discuss options and possible long-term consequences with doctors and surgeons, say former patients. Their diagnosis was invariably followed by a rapid sequence of events leading to rapid treatment. This suits some men. But others can feel railroaded in retrospect. They follow the advice – and invariably the professional interest – of the consultant they see because they perceive that time is of the essence. But after the treatment, and living with some of its long-term consequences, many wonder why no one really explored with them the quality of life issues related to each treatment. Would just watching and waiting have been a better option, given the fact that many prostate cancers are slow growing?

'I should have discussed what I was feeling before the surgery'

Among those with regrets is Ken Mastris, a board member of the European Cancer Patient Coalition. In hindsight, he says, he wishes he had asked for more information about alternatives when his surgeon recommended radical prostatectomy. 'At that stage I didn't know anything, not even what the prostate did, and I didn't question what he said. When you first get a diagnosis, your first thought is to get rid of the cancer out of your body. But I should have discussed what I was feeling before the surgery.'

 Another man, living with long-term continence and erection problems following surgery, told me that he had discovered through long personal experience of prostate cancer and conversations with men in similar circumstances that there was no one 'truth' about best treatment, best approach, best outcome. Yet doctors suggest there is, on the basis of very partial knowledge about outcomes. 'Medicine is very bad at presenting the fact that they don't know what the consequences will be for you', he said.

> Everyone wants things to be clean cut, but you just don't know what will happen in the long term in your case. They tell you this and that might happen, but only you will find out what happens for you. I think there needs to be more honesty about this, to give men greater opportunity to think about what's right for them in the long run.

Evidence of psychological effects

For some men, treatment brings few long-term side effects and they live a good quality life. Others adjust and manage to live a relatively normal life even though they have these issues.

And some don't. The long-term physical consequences of prostate cancer treatment can be intertwined with worry, regret, anxiety and depression. Some men blame themselves for choosing the treatment they did. The corrosive influence of this should not be underestimated. A recent study found that 15 years after treatment, 15 per cent of men regretted deciding on surgery for prostate cancer and 16.6 per cent regretted deciding on radiotherapy. The regret tended to increase with time (Hoffman *et al.* 2017).

The psychological impacts associated with long-term treatment consequences go far wider. A review of studies published in 2017 concluded that men experience physical, psychological and social changes after prostatectomy, and that their perceptions of masculinity are affected (Kong, Deatrick and Bradway 2017). Men often described prostate surgery as 'life-changing'. And although they recognised the trade-off between survival and post-operative complications, long-term effects such as erectile dysfunction often caused them more distress than the potential return of the disease itself. Another review concluded that men's sense of masculinity was invariably diminished after treatment (Alexis and Worsley 2018).

Exactly how many men are coping and how many are not? Currently, it's hard to tell. One recent study found that 36.5 per cent of men who had radical prostatectomy saw sexual functioning as a 'big problem' 24 months after treatment. Perhaps most significantly, 17 per cent of men reported moderate to severe levels of anxiety and 10 per cent moderate to severe levels of depression two years after treatment (Watson *et al.* 2015).

There's evidence that the consequence of these long-term mental health effects can be extreme. A raft of studies published in the mid-2000s demonstrated that the suicide rate is significantly higher among cancer patients than the general population. One study indicated that it is twice as prevalent, and remained elevated for 15 years after a cancer diagnosis. Higher suicide rates were associated with being male, white or unmarried (Sharma 2008).

More recently, research has spotlighted just how high the suicide rate is for men with cancers of the male genitourinary system, which make up around 40 per cent of cancers in men in the UK, and where treatment often brings consequences for continence and sexual function. A major study led by the University of Birmingham[1] has found that men with cancers of the bladder, prostate, penis, testes and kidney are five times more likely to take their own lives than the general population. The rate for cancer patients generally is three times that of the general population.

This is not a matter of impulsive, desperate acts straight after diagnosis. The research showed that the average (median) time from diagnosis to suicide for patients with prostate cancer was about 28 months. Dr Mehran Afshar from St George's Hospital London, who wrote the study, has pointed out that the particular symptoms that can follow treatment for these kinds of cancer can alter personalities and lead to relationship problems, anxiety, depression and post-traumatic stress disorder. A lot of men become very desperate.

Men talking about tough experiences

Yet there's a strange disconnect between such research and personal accounts from patients. When do we see men talking

---

1   See https://eau18.uroweb.org/major-study-shows-x5-greater-suicide-rate-
    in-patients-with-urological-cancers/

about their experiences of these issues? Honest personal accounts of life after prostate cancer – of any male cancer – are as rare as hen's teeth. Even at conferences about prostate cancer, I have found that men rarely talk about the detail of their own experiences and anxieties, just the issues.

I have learned as much about what life is like with and after prostate cancer by talking to relatives who, like myself, have had to live with the day-to-day changes and stresses that treatment can bring. They talk about parents or spouses just getting on with it, but seeing the small signs of disquiet: embarrassment at accidents, leakages or frequent toilet visits, a weary awareness that they have become simultaneously childlike and old.

It sounds minor, but it's stuck with me how much my dad hated being unable to have hot baths during his radiotherapy because he was worried that everyone would think he smelled. I remember him starting to shuffle around more after treatment, as if his confidence in himself had been knocked. Most of all, I remember a new distracted, worried look. 'Will this never end?' it seemed to say.

Of course, these were just signs I picked up: Dad never wanted to share what he was going through with me. But when men do talk openly and honestly about the experiences of living after prostate cancer, it is curiously affecting.

'Options which doctors regard as successful just aren't viewed in the same way by the men'

One man I talked to is one of those who looks back with regret, most of all because he had little idea how treatment might affect his sex life. The problem, he said, was that doctors always want to be positive about what they do. So although the possibilities of side effects are discussed, they are presented as fixable – at least as far as the medic is concerned.

They tell you that if you have erection problems after the surgery, there are things you can do, like take a little blue pill. But actually, in real life, it hasn't helped me much. My wife and I find it very difficult to plan sex in advance – it just doesn't suit our lives – but that's what you have to do if you use Viagra because it takes a while to work. So that's not a solution. It's the same thing with pads. They're presented as a solution to incontinence after treatment. But they're not: they're just a way of keeping things less messy. I find this very frustrating, and I'm aware that options which doctors regard as successful just aren't viewed in the same way by the men who are living through it.

The side effects after treatment affect your life more than is often thought, or described in studies. In the end, it's up to you – and your partner – to find your own solutions in order to achieve the best possible quality of life. The medical profession needs to have a greater understanding of these aspects.

His view about the difference between medical and patient perspectives is backed up by studies. Research published in the *European Journal of Cancer* (Gravis *et al.* 2014) revealed a stark mismatch between doctors' assessment of side effects and the patients they had treated for metastatic prostate cancer. It found that physicians systematically under-report patients' symptoms after hormone therapy, with patients generally reporting double the severity of side effects. Six months after treatment, patients' evaluation of the impact of joint pain, sexual dysfunction, weight loss and urinary dysfunction was at least four times greater than that of health professionals' evaluation.

Just getting on with it

It would be wrong to suggest that all men are struggling on silently with terrible after-effects. I have spoken to men who have been treated for prostate cancer who are positive about their experiences. Yes, things are different, but the support of family and close friends makes things workable, and brings new outlooks on life and a different kind of closeness. You just work with what you've got, and take the best from it, they say.

Some of these viewpoints are represented in an excellent series of video interviews with men talking about prostate cancer experiences, published online by the charity Prostate Cancer UK. I would recommend the videos to anyone involved in healthcare. While acknowledging the significant problems they have faced, the interviewees are generally emphatic that men can get through them, and that supportive family and friends are key. At the same time, most also allude to some of the intense internal struggles of life after treatment.

Bruce, who was diagnosed in 2009, speaks of how his ongoing hormone therapy leaves him bloated and tearful. 'One of the worst things is having man boobs', he says. 'You just have to accept you need bigger jeans.' His advice? Dig deep.

Ally had 36 radiotherapy treatments, plus hormone therapy, after diagnosis in 2010. The worst side effects were tiredness and suddenly needing to go to the toilet. He still gets tired, but makes the effort to go out. He advises: '100 per cent and more, stay positive.'

Paul has had incontinence and erectile dysfunction since having a radical prostatectomy in 2009. It does, he acknowledges, 'make you think about who you are as a man', but his wife has been very supportive. The important thing, he says, is to be positive and adjust your life. 'You adapt and then you make that adaptation as good as possible.'

You will note a common theme here: the importance of staying positive, of defying what is happening to you and getting on with life, the quality that might once have been called having a 'stiff upper lip'.

Men and the 'coping' question

This determined outlook is not unique to people who have had prostate cancer. The need to 'stay positive' is commonly recommended by and to people with cancer – and, indeed, by many lifestyle gurus. For some, it helps; for others, it doesn't – in fact, for some people the pressure to feel something they can't makes things worse.

But the frequency with which men talk about the need to 'just get on with life' does raise two issues. First, it brings up the predictable and thorny subject of how men deal with difficult situations, and whether by just carrying on and not talking about their sadness, worries and resentments they store them up and suffer the mental health consequences, sometimes with catastrophic consequences.

Second, it raises the important question of what it is about the new world men are thrown into by urological cancers that makes it so difficult to deal with. Is there something particular about the male cancer experience that distinguishes it from the more general cancer experience? Could understanding this better help drive the ways support services develop?

The talking issue

Let's not get bogged down in the first question. Bemoaning the fact that men don't open up about their problems – 'If only men were more like women' – gets us nowhere. All men and all women are on a spectrum of emotional intelligence and personality type: some find it easier to talk than others, and there's only so much you can do to change that. Of course, giving everyone the opportunity to talk is crucial – and if health service providers were more skilled at making space for those opportunities 'after' cancer as well as during it, it would make an enormous difference to many people living with long-term effects.

Many men do find talking therapy – in informal groups, with counsellors or psychotherapists – very beneficial. More and more men are attending private and NHS therapy sessions when they experience physical or mental ill health. They welcome the opportunity to throw off the shackles of traditional male roles, to show emotion and not feel judged if they reveal vulnerability. The anonymity and confidentiality of such sessions is important. The male suicide charity CALM has pointed out that it's a myth that men don't want to talk about their feelings: they often simply don't want to share their problems with family, friends and colleagues (Doward 2015).

There's also some evidence that men open up extremely successfully when they're in groups of men who have had similar experiences. Psychologist Martin Seager, for example, has said that in single-sex groups men can be very blokey one minute, and talk about something extremely painful the next. Alone in a room together, they can be like soldiers in combat, supporting and caring for each other (Daubney 2015).

But the fact will always remain that many men don't want to talk. Many cope by just getting on with it – trying to put the bad stuff at the back of their minds and asserting normality. That's the way that many men in the Prostate Cancer UK videos were coping. We can say this 'plough-through-it' attitude has damaging consequences, but for some it works, and even for those who need more, it's still one type of coping mechanism. It's not a fault.

The disorientating world of urology

So what about the specific experience of urological cancers? Concepts of masculinity are obviously at stake here. There's also something immediately difficult about the most intimate organs and functions being subjected to intimate scientific scrutiny because they are 'a problem'. They are suddenly public, even if the 'public' is just your healthcare team. This clearly applies to cancers affecting women too.

But when faced with long-term problems of potency and continence, how easy is it for men to regain their sense of ownership? It sounds terrible to say, but for many people, the very word 'urology' evokes thoughts of bad smells, leakages and old age. And if those associations are there through years of clinic visits, how much do they gradually wear away at self-esteem? How much does it affect who you feel you are?

'I still feel awkward in this waiting room', said Nick, a man I talked to while waiting for a urological appointment.

> It's not who I feel I am. It sounds stupid, but I don't want to tell people about my treatment or its effects because I worry what they'll think of me. Here I am, 60, married, but I still like to think of myself as not unappealing to women. It's not exactly dashing, is it, running off to the toilet. It's the same with my friends. I feel if I told them, they'd somehow think I was a bit sad, old.

I, like Nick, was temporarily thrown into the world that my father had been forced to be part of at a similar age, when I was investigated for prostate cancer and subjected to a biopsy. I dipped into the urological universe of needles, biopsies, sample jars, weak tea, overused toilets, cold hands, rubber gloves, lubricants, and information sheets that don't tell you anything you want to know.

The whole thing, which dragged on due to unpleasant side effects from the biopsy, didn't feel very 'me'. It felt old, dependent – something you're reluctant to tell people about. I'm pretty sure that everyone else feels the same way.

The onset of any illness or disability brings a journey into alien territory. But for men with urological problems, there's something isolating about the associations. It's about the cold medicalisation of the parts of the body that are meant to be associated with pleasure; it's about fear of age; it's about social embarrassment; it's about perceptions of masculinity.

The problem for men who are living for years with the after-effects of prostate cancer is that whatever the cancer outcome, these weird feelings and insecurities continue. Sometimes they never go away. Some men are left with an ever-withering image of themselves as energetic and virile. Why this should be has as much to do with society's expectations as men's emotional fragility.

30 years on – who's looking at the bigger picture?

These are complex and difficult issues. But the long-term negative effects of treatment for male urological cancers clearly interweave with the physical and psychological. All too often the approach of health services is to offer a specific solution to a specific problem – prescribing continence pads, for example, or suggesting counselling for depression – without paying attention to the bigger picture. What can be done to make men feel less medicalised, to make patient perceptions of what they are experiencing more real – and more of a priority – to clinicians?

I don't want to suggest in any way that men with prostate cancer, or men with cancer generally, are the only ones who experience issues with identity, sexuality, gender, or self-worth as a result of cancer and its treatments. This is clearly not the case. But the statistics on male cancers and mental health alone suggest that something important is going on.

Looking back over the past 30 years, I am astounded at some of the advances in prostate cancer diagnosis, monitoring and treatment. I'm fairly sure that if Dad had received a prompt diagnosis today we could have expected him to live 20 years or more, rather than the five he actually had. But at the same time, I also wonder how much has changed once treatment ends. If Dad had received curative treatment, what consequences would he be left with? How would he have coped?

I'd like to think that there is more long-term support today; that physicians are better tuned into their patients' feelings; that there's less bellicosity about cure; that it's not all down to families and just 'getting on with life' any more. I'd like to think that men with cancer embark on their treatment decisions forewarned and forearmed, so that they know they're facing an uncertain future but that they won't have to face it alone and unprepared. But I listen to the stories and look at the research, and I'm not so sure.

Simon Crompton is an award-winning writer and editor, journalist and communications consultant specialising in health, science and social affairs. He has a special interest in cancer and men's health is a regular contributor to *Cancer World* magazine and has written for *The Times* since 1998.

www.simoncrompton.com

@simoncrompton2

CHAPTER 9

THE WAY FORWARD

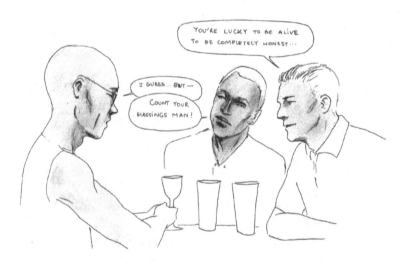

Greater recognition and acceptance of the long-term effects of cancer is vital

The strong message of this book is that *there needs to be much greater acceptance and recognition of the long-term effects of cancer, both psychological and physical.*

In a sense, this is a message that is for the benefit of us all, too, since cancer is now often considered a common and chronic condition, if you survive it. Throughout the world, increasing numbers are diagnosed with one form of cancer or another, and it makes sense to say that as survival rates improve, more and more of us will be affected by some version of cancer's long-term effects. If we, ourselves, are not affected, most of us already know people who are. That's how widespread this problem is. It is therefore high time that the huge issue of cancer's long-term effects ceases to be perceived as a niche problem and starts to be understood for what it is, a potentially vast one. As Professor Smith in Chapter 7 highlighted, we don't even have a word for it yet, but there will soon be an epidemic we can't handle if we don't recognise and start to deal with it now.

I also hope it is clear that, for the sake of all those with long-term effects, and cancer care in general, *it is vital that we urgently*:

- examine the myriad of reasons why these effects are not often adequately recognised or attended to
- challenge our own and others' entrenched thinking and beliefs about cancer and about how life should be after a cancer diagnosis
- recognise and accept that significant numbers endure these effects, rather than assuming that these are the problems of a minority who survive cancer
- recognise and accept the nature of these effects
- recognise the negative psychological effects of lack of recognition on those coping with long-term effects
- create and promote more initiatives to help those struggling with long-term effects (see Ben Parker's comments below about government initiatives and the need to implement them, such as the Recovery Package)
- recognise that these initiatives need to be driven by those who are willing to try to understand the predicament of those enduring these effects and are prepared to listen to what is needed from those affected

- implement these initiatives
- commission more qualitative research on the psychological impact of the long-term effects of cancer, led by researchers who have both relevant expertise and an open-minded and non-entrenched approach. The involvement of researchers with insider knowledge is also key to the generation of accurate data.

The need to think outside the 'received wisdom' box

The above can only happen if we are able and willing to be open to different ways of thinking about the long-term effects of cancer. We might then be able to consider new ways of supporting those affected.

Some questions we could very usefully ask, whether we are health professionals working in the cancer field or others wanting to understand and help, include:

- Is it at all possible to have a diagnosis of cancer and not be heavily traumatised by it?
- Is it at all possible to have a diagnosis of cancer and not be terrified of it returning?
- Is it at all possible to be treated for cancer and not suffer any side effects of treatment, either shorter, longer term, or both?
- Is there enough general understanding of the impact of a diagnosis of cancer on an individual?
- Do existing systems, structures and common practices within medicine lend themselves to over-treatment of some cancers in some patients?
- Is there adequate information given to people about the treatment options available to them?

- Is there enough respect for and understanding and acceptance of people who don't want to undergo all the treatments they are offered?
- Are patients given adequate choices about their treatments?
- Is as much emphasis placed on the psychological impact of cancer as on its physical impact?
- Is the commonality of experience among cancer patients accepted enough, both the psychological and the physical?
- Do we have adequate understanding of the psychology of trauma and specifically, of cancer?

Additionally, *it is very important to recognise that a person's experience of cancer and its longer-term effects will be affected by a number of factors*, including:

- their prognosis
- the treatments they have had or are enduring
- the reactions of those around them; for example, family, friends, healthcare professionals
- how well those around them understand the psychological and physical impacts of long-term problems
- the amount of support they have available to them, both practical and emotional.

External factors will impact those affected, for example:

- the Western world's continuing understandable, but extreme, fear of cancer
- cancer's continuing historical legacy as a disease that always kills its host
- the pejorative language we use in English, for example, 'it's like a cancer in our society'

- the covert way in which we talk about and deal with
  death in Western society
- the limitations of medical science
- the degree of support that is available from government
  for those suffering long-term effects from cancer,
  financial and otherwise.

For healthcare professionals
working with cancer patients

I well know that working in healthcare, whether in the public
or private sector, is extremely hard work and that there are
many factors militating against offering patients the kind
of treatment and general support we would like to offer,
particularly so in the public sector. I also know what great
work many in healthcare do and how much patients benefit
from the untiring commitment of a wide range of healthcare
professionals' input.

Nevertheless, the questions below are important professional development questions for all of us, and there is still
much we can offer patients that will improve the quality of
care we offer them, in spite of all the constraints on us. These
are not meant to imply criticism in any way. They are tough
questions, but are intended to benefit staff and patients alike.

Questions you could ask yourself:

- How aware am I of the problem of long-term effects of
  cancer?
- What do I think or feel about the whole issue of long-
  term effects? For example, do I agree that this is really a
  problem? Do I think the problems are overstated in this
  book? Generally?
- What do I think about the author's dual perspective
  approach in this book? Does it add value or not?

- What did I think about Chapter 2 and the reasons that were suggested for why people tend to sweep the long-term effects of cancer under the carpet?
- Did I learn anything?
- On a scale of 1–10, if 10 is open-minded about the issue of cancer's long-term effects and 1 is sceptical, where would I honestly put myself on that scale?
- Do I believe in the long-term psychological effects of cancer more than the physical, or vice versa, or do I believe in both?
- How did I react to Chapter 7, where the doctors and nurse were outlining their clinical experience, thoughts and feelings about long-term effects? Did I learn anything?
- How well did my training equip me for dealing with patients with cancer, particularly a while after diagnosis?
- How did I react to Chapters 3, 4 and 5? Did I learn anything?
- Are these questions irritating me? If yes, why is that?
- How do I feel about cancer generally; for example, how do I deal with my fear of getting it myself? (If you have had a diagnosis already, see the separate section below.)
- Do my thoughts and feelings about cancer impact on my work with my patients? How?
- How do I deal with the stress of my job? Do I ask for support? Admit when I'm stressed? Does it feel like I'm failing if I think about asking for help?
- What support or training would be helpful to me at work, regarding cancer's long-term effects?
- Have I ever spoken to anyone with long-term effects and really listened to what they have to say?

For those who suffer longer-term from cancer

I hope this book has offered you support that has been valuable and that you can recognise your situation, or aspects of it, within it. I am sure you have picked up from what I have written that I have problems with long-term effects myself, so I understand, from the inside, how hard life can be.

Although this is not a self-help book, I have tried to give anyone coping with long-term effects, whatever they may be, some strategies for improving their quality of life and some general support, and, not least, validation of the complex nature of cancer's effects.

In summary:

- My biggest message in this book, to those coping with cancer's effects, be they more or less extreme, is to allow yourself to validate how you feel in the face of others ignoring your predicament, and/or their ignorance of it. *What you experience is real*, no matter what they say or don't say.

- No matter what version of the long-term effects you are coping with, spanning degrees of disability with no recurrence to recurrence and living in the knowledge that your life may or will end soon, while there are clearly vast differences between these situations, one thing many of us need is *greater recognition of what cancer's effects do or have done* to us.

- For those who survive beyond diagnosis, across the whole spectrum of possible diagnoses, I have spoken in this book about the benefits of speaking out about these problems in order to educate others, as well as the possible benefits to the individual 'sufferer' if they do speak out. Not least, *our quality of life can be improved by risking speaking out*. I hope I have also made it clear that not everyone will want to speak out and that that is fine, too. It is an individual choice.

- As death approaches, if those who are very sick speak out, their words can certainly be powerfully educational for others, should anyone in this situation wish to or choose to (and clearly there is no right or wrong way to cope with approaching death). Someone who decided to speak out was Dr Kate Granger,[1] who died of cancer in July 2016. She achieved a huge amount in the years following her diagnosis in 2011 in the field of cancer care. She did so by challenging myths around cancer, as well as many other aspects of patient care, from her dual perspective of medical doctor and a woman with terminal cancer. Her powerful words live on beyond her death and are a salutary reminder to all of us *to listen, re-think our approach and take heed.*

- Recognising the history within medicine and healthcare generally, that militates against the acceptance of our problems after cancer, the 'you should be over it in a year' school of thought, can be helpful, too. It's worth remembering that *healthcare professionals are usually not trained in any aspect of the long-term effects of cancer.*
  - Often enough, they are ignorant of the effects rather than unwilling to listen, although obviously, there are those who are entrenched in their positions and who are not willing or able to consider anything outside this version.

The following strategies can help those enduring cancer's long-term effects:

---

1   See https://drkategranger.wordpress.com

- Telling people how you feel can be very empowering and can have a positive effect, both on you and on others.
- Standing up to those who belittle your suffering can be empowering.
- Laying down boundaries with others can also be very useful; for example, 'I am not going to do such and such anymore, because doing so is making my life harder.'
- Asking yourself how much you collude in a version that goes 'I shouldn't complain' or 'these long-term problems are in my mind' can be helpful.

For those who are both healthcare professionals and long-term sufferers

If you, like me, are both a healthcare professional and someone who has had a diagnosis of cancer and suffers longer term, there might be elements in both sections above that resonate with you.

Key for me, at any rate, is recognising how much the medical model approach to healthcare militates against the acceptance of me as both a psychologist and cancer patient. My psychologist voice is seldom well received when I combine it with my patient concerns. And the difficulty we have in healthcare accepting both voices coming from the same individual is one that needs tackling.

Just recognising that these problems accepting the dual identity of patients exist, especially so in healthcare, can help me cope. If I remind myself in any given situation that I am finding hard that the problem probably doesn't emanate from within me, that it is an institutional problem, this can take the pressure off me.

In my case, obviously, I speak out about the issues I have raised in this book, through writing and other media. While this is not everyone's preference, even 'speaking out to yourself' in private can help.

It would, of course, be wonderful if more health professionals who have had a diagnosis of cancer and are living with its effects long-term would also speak out from their dual perspective. I recognise it can be hard to do so, for the reasons outlined in this book; for example, fear of being judged, pathologised and even losing our jobs. And in a sense, attitudes within healthcare towards those of us who have this dual perspective need to change first, so people can feel freed up to openly be both healthcare professionals and those suffering longer term, rather than either one or the other. The question overall is, how do we change attitudes, practices, etc.? This is a high, potentially hazardous, mountain to climb...

For family, friends and colleagues

- Being open to even part of what is suggested in this chapter will very likely be welcomed by your family member/friend/colleague suffering the long-term effects of cancer.
- Just recognising that long-term effects exist and can cause varying degrees of problems can be a huge help to those coping with these effects. If you are able to acknowledge this openly with a family member/friend/ colleague, this might well be welcomed.
- Asking those concerned how you can help them, no matter what context you know them in, is very supportive. If they hesitate to say anything, asking again at some point might be welcomed. I know, from personal experience, that people can be reticent about saying what they need. Often, we are so used to coping alone or in silence that we struggle to ask, but this

doesn't mean we don't want help. Next time we are asked, we might come up with a request.

- Recognising how scared the majority of us are of recurrence is very important and this fear is bound to affect how we behave. We may or may not want to talk about it, but it will be there in the background, foreground or somewhere in-between, depending on what is going on in our lives.
- Recognising how the wider context, mentioned above, affects those coping longer term with cancer's fall-out is imperative; for example, how the collective beliefs of society at large about cancer impact on those enduring long-term effects is important.

The current situation in the UK regarding support for those with long-term effects

The situation concerning support for those suffering the long-term effects of cancer in the UK today has been mentioned at various points in this book.

Macmillan Cancer Support, along with others working in cancer care and healthcare generally, are leading the way in trying to make sure government initiatives are implemented. Ben Parker, Senior Public Affairs Officer at Macmillan, sums up the situation as follows:

With more people than ever living with cancer and its potentially life-changing implications, it's vital that the right support exists for people after they have finished treatment.

With a wide range of possible physical, emotional and attitudinal barriers that people can face after they have finished treatment for cancer, it's critically important that the Government and the NHS adapts to better meet these needs. This is why Macmillan has continued to push for the implementation of initiatives such as the Recovery Package. The Recovery Package is a way of working that aims to ensure that the changing needs of people living with cancer are identified and addressed, from diagnosis through treatment to recovery, so that their care is person-centred and their health and wellbeing needs are supported. The concept of the Recovery Package was developed and tested by the National Cancer Survivorship Initiative (2008–2013) – a partnership of Macmillan Cancer Support, the Department of Health and NHS England. It was subsequently adopted as Government policy in 2015, with the stated commitment that everyone with a cancer diagnosis would have access to the Recovery Package by 2020.

In a nutshell, and as Ben emphasises, 'It is welcome that the Government [in the UK] has committed to implementing the Recovery Package, but more work is needed before it is a reality on the ground for everyone with cancer.'

A final word from me

And as I end, I echo what Ben says, that much more awareness is needed if we are ever going to offer better support to the growing numbers living with cancer's long-term effects.

I also echo the words of Dr Evans, the oncologist from Chapter 7, who said that it is only through the success of the cure that you start to see the long-term consequences of the treatment. The job of work now is to 'look and see', rather than turning a blind eye to the resultant problems people endure.

And now I rest my case, in the hope that others will increasingly take up the mantle and dare to tread where many fear to go, and, in the process, effect change in this complex and troublesome area. I can only hope.

MITZI'S STORY: ANAL AND BREAST CANCER

Mitzi Blennerhassett was diagnosed with two cancers, the first one, anal cancer, in 1990, and the second, breast cancer, in 1997. The following is her exposé of her life since both diagnoses, starting with anal cancer. It is a shocking series of accounts, but sadly, she is not alone in her experiences. It's tempting, even for me, to tell myself that Mitzi's story is rare, but unfortunately, having spoken to so many people about life after cancer, I know there are significant numbers of others experiencing similar symptoms, including me.

The recurring themes throughout her testimony are 'nobody told me this would happen' and 'nobody much has listened to me when I have tried to tell them what I am suffering'. These are common themes for those of us suffering long-term effects.

Fortunately, there has been a modicum of help for her, but Mitzi has had to speak out and push for it. Not everyone is able to do this. Even so, she needs much more help and support than she is getting. The following is her story to date.

First diagnosis: anal cancer

'I felt I was being tortured'

I had carcinoma of the anal canal in 1990 when I was aged 50: I was told the side effects of treatment would be nausea, sickness, diarrhoea and wind. Nobody mentioned the long-term effects.

Some side effects did not disappear, so have become 'long-term effects'

Bowel problems

Cancer treatments saved my life but bowel problems such as urgency, lack of control, violent spasm, wind and acute pain persisted and worsened over time, and still have a significant impact on my quality of life.

Twenty-eight years after cancer treatment, my bowel still tears and bleeds; the medication of a mini-enema exacerbates pain. Defecation can be a terrifying ordeal lasting over two hours, during which time symptoms will include bleeding, severe sweating and nausea, while weakness and shakiness particularly affect my legs, which feel semi-paralysed.

Midline lymphoedema (swelling from abdominal fluid due to damaged lymphatic system or lymph nodes)

I had never heard of lymphoedema and nobody mentioned this possible side effect during or after treatment. Despite the diagnosis of NHS radiation-induced lymphoedema, I was not able to get any satisfactory treatment until 2005, when I underwent a formal complaint. Although a six-week intensive manual lymphatic drainage (MLD) course commissioned by the then Primary Care Trust (PCT) in 2005 was monitored at the beginning and end and pronounced successful with 3L fluid lost, I have not been able to access a further similar course of treatment and daily self-management is insufficient for my needs: despite three years of heroic attempts by my GP, each of her requests to the Clinical Commissioning Group (CCG) Individual Funding Request Panel have been declined. The GP said there was little point in writing again as 'nobody is getting anything because the CCG hasn't any money!' Bizarrely, the CCG suggested lymphoedema clinics which (a) only treated arm lymphoedema or (b) happened to be the very clinic from which I was discharged after being told they could not give even short MLD treatments in future, except to new patients. Then NHS support panty-hose garments (regularly supplied since diagnosis) were withdrawn. I was advised to buy my own, at a cost of approximately £50 per garment.

Osteoporosis

I was diagnosed with osteoporosis in 2011. After a few months, a spinal fracture occurred as I bent down, followed by excruciating pain from muscle spasm. I managed to drive to the GP surgery by keeping my back rigid and pressing the top of my shoulders against the car seat, but it was agony. I was invited to touch my toes and perhaps this achievement (although causing great pain) led the GP to say it was 'just pulled muscles'. Various exercises were recommended, but they simply exacerbated pain. Months later, an X-ray confirmed a wedge fracture at T11 and I began taking bisphosphonate medication, Alondronate, along with calcium and vitamin D tablets.

I stopped taking the pills after two years, as the side effects were adversely affecting my quality of life and there seemed little evidence of efficacy.

Second diagnosis: breast cancer

I had a diagnosis of breast cancer in 1997. Surgery (lumpectomy) was followed by radiotherapy and Tamoxifen.

I was in the middle of a Fine Art BA (Honours) degree course when I found a breast lump and immediately went to my GP. Despite its hard, pea-like structure and my previous history of cancer, he assured me it was a harmless fibroadenoma. 'Anyway, the mobile mammography unit will be around in the next month or two', he said. 'That will sort you out, one way or another.' I knew mammography alone was not appropriate for diagnosing breast cancer. Macmillan Spotlight Series and NHS Improving Outcomes referral guidelines indicated that my age and my cancer history, plus the position of the lump and the fact that I had been taking HRT for 10 years, meant immediate referral was necessary. The referral five months later was thanks to a cervical cytology clinic doctor who examined my breasts and advised the GP of his findings. (He still took two weeks before writing to the breast consultant, saying he felt sure this was not necessary, 'but she has taken herself off to a clinic...')

Cording

After breast surgery (lumpectomy) I exercised as advised, but experienced excruciating pain from armpit to nipple, as if a cord adhering to my flesh was being pulled out. I could not lift my arm above horizontal and noticed with horror that my armpit was divided into two hollows. I contacted the breast clinic and spoke to the surgeon but was disappointed that he refused to recognise this as a problem and, even without seeing me, stated that it would be fine. Feeling abandoned, I rang a national cancer support charity who put me in touch with a physiotherapist at a well-known London cancer hospital; she said it sounded like 'cording', a well-known post-surgical condition, but one many surgeons failed to acknowledge. (Did they see this as some sort of failure, I wondered?) She advised me that I'd need many weeks of physiotherapy with strong painkillers, and my GP arranged this.

Cording responded to physiotherapy but I still experience occasional cramp-like pains across the lower part of my breast and have hard, tender breast lumps. There are also similar lumps in my other breast and rib tenderness, probably due to 'scatter' radiation.

Tamoxifen

The drug Tamoxifen affected me so badly I had to take a year out of college and commute from a BA Honours to the shorter BA. Side effects included extreme hot flushes, sleeplessness, nausea and lack of stamina that left me too unwell to cope with daily chores. Itchy skin symptoms worsened; my eyebrows looked moth-eaten and frequent vaginal bleeding resulted in annual hospitalisation for uterine examination under general anaesthetic (G/A). I discovered this would routinely include a dilation and curettage of my womb, although patients were not informed about this. Most women on my ward were suffering the same symptoms from the same cause as me. I stopped taking Tamoxifen after two years, as I felt so unwell. Also, I did not want to become a 'permanent patient', having to undergo annual check-ups under G/A and all that entailed. Hot flushes continued for years, and although reduced, they still occur frequently as my body is unable to regulate heat; my comfort zone is very narrow.

Bronchiectasis

This is a long-term, progressive condition where the airways are abnormally widened and lung secretions are not cleared in the normal way via cilia. It is different from, but related to, chronic obstructive pulmonary disease (COPD).

Although the oncologist explained that radiotherapy for breast cancer in 1997 might damage a tiny piece of lung, I was not affected by shortness of breath or other lung problems until 2007, when acute pain developed in the front of my chest. When I breathed in it felt as if my lung was ripping. Most days, I had fits of coughing that lasted two hours and could no longer walk up the slightest slope without stopping to get my breath. My GP thought it was asthma, but the inhalers she prescribed did not alleviate the condition. At a routine hospital check-up several months later, I mentioned the cough to my breast oncologist and after investigations was diagnosed with bronchiectasis, a condition unknown to me.

Having bronchiectasis limits my social life as I am prone to lung infections and at particular risk of complications from pneumonia and influenza; visits from grandchildren, with their coughs and colds, have become mixed blessings; and ordinary head colds often become chest infections with resultant massive build-up of mucus in my lungs, causing frequent, distressing (and disgusting) coughing and choking sessions. Each of these 'exacerbations' causes further lung damage.

Overall effects

Relationships

Marriage breakdown and divorce followed two years after the first cancer in 1990, due partly to over-sensitivity and lowered tolerance levels (allodynia) following cancer. Treatment side effects also meant sexual intercourse was difficult and painful. Bowel problems can blight close relationships too!

Inability to work

Frailty and treatment side effects after cancer in 1990 prevented me from returning to part-time secretarial and reception work at a rural, single-handed GP practice, and the second cancer in 1997 added to my difficulties. However, I was fortunate that voluntary work offered opportunities that could fit around my fatigue. Locally, I helped to set up and run a cancer support group and became a member of the Community Health Council, while medical Royal Colleges' user involvement groups and other national organisations gave me a voice to influence change.

My writing ability as a health campaigner and author is now limited, due to pain and other side effects mentioned above.

Financial burdens

No one explained that I might be eligible for disability benefits after cancer in 1990, and it was only after I left my husband, two years later, that I applied for state benefits. Access was delayed, allegedly because I was doing a part-time educational course, which meant my son and I lived for four months without any income.

Psychological effects

Long-term effects of cancer treatments tended to lower my self-esteem, but the respect and inclusiveness shown by some health professionals in user involvement groups enabled me to influence change nationally, and this boosted my morale. Slimness due to cancer treatments was an unexpected bonus, but midline lymphoedema was a shocking unexpected blow; it changed my body image and destroyed my confidence ('what else had they not warned me about?'). Although I came to terms with NHS treatment-induced lymphoedema, it has been depressing to realise I cannot access another effective MLD course for this progressive disease. I feel abandoned by the NHS.

Long-term effects such as pain can bring back unwanted memories of cancer treatments, causing me to re-live events. Life should be especially precious after surviving two cancers, but daily self-management routines, necessary to control side effects, contribute to a lowered quality of life. I sometimes have to remind myself that there are plenty of people worse off than me in order to get through the day.

Paternalism should have died in the 20th century. However well meant, medical paternalism during cancer treatment in 1990 eroded trust. Since then, I have been fortunate to work alongside like-minded, dedicated health professionals: shared aims and mutual respect has allowed trust to blossom. With the advent of patient empowerment, partnership working and the drive towards patient autonomy has come much positive change. Sometimes, however, the balance of power in a doctor-patient relationship can still be lacking.

The need to raise awareness

Of course, I am grateful that NHS treatments saved my life. However, lack of shared information, especially about potential side effects, meant I was treated as a less than competent adult, with adverse psychological and physiological consequences. I wondered if doctors simply could not acknowledge that their treatments caused harm.

More awareness is needed about cancer treatment side effects: drugs to alleviate those effects may adversely affect other health conditions. One medical condition may affect another: the weight of lymphoedema fluid in my abdomen severely exacerbates pain from spinal arthritis (plus the T11 fracture, allodynia, etc.), which should be taken into account when doctors decide whether or not to grant individualised access to MLD treatment for lymphoedema.

We need greater use of patients and patient speakers in medical education so that health professionals understand the consequences of paternalism, and why honesty and compassion are vital to modern health services.

In order to make informed choices before consenting to cancer treatments people need full information about:

- potential late and long-term effects, however rare
- methods of prevention (where this is possible)
- quality of life issues.

One of the standards in the General Medical Council's booklet,[1] 'Good Medical Practice', is 'give patients the information they want or need to know in a way they can understand' (Domain 3: Communicate Effectively, No. 32, p.16).

It is not enough to treat the disease

Cancer patients who experience long-term, treatment-induced side effects need ongoing support and access to services that can alleviate those conditions. NHS treatment for side effects should be lifelong and available nationwide, instead of varying according to postcode.

Tips for coping with lymphoedema

Anne Vadgama, an experienced MLD therapist, suggests the following to help manage the condition, no matter what the cause.

---

1   www.gmc-uk.org/ethical-guidance/ethical-guidance-for-doctors/good-medical-practice/domain-3---communication-partnership-and-teamwork

Clothing

- Clothing should be loose and comfortable, without bra straps, socks, etc. cutting in.
- Try to stay cool in summer, as heat can aggravate oedema.
- Lymphoedema hosiery (LH) only works well if comfortable.
- LH should be worn all day, while active, in the early days, until the lymphoedema is stable, then slowly and carefully experiment with cutting down the length of time LH is worn.
- LH should be worn when travelling, especially when flying and seated for lengthy periods in cars and other forms of transport, including when sitting at desks and other seated events.
- Genital lymphoedema can be helped by wearing tight Lycra cycling shorts.

Diet

- Diet should be healthy, with a minimum of processed foods that often have additives, preservatives and hidden salts and sugars.
- Fluid uptake should be regular to assist flushing the system.

Exercise

- Follow specific exercises for your type of oedema, and adhere to the recommended frequency and repetitions – sometimes more is not more!
- Any other sport and/or physical activity should be undertaken within your capacity and comfort zone,

starting slowly and in small amounts, building up as you feel comfortable and not over- or under-exerting yourself.

- Deep abdominal breathing acts as a pump for all the lymphatics of the lower body.
- All muscular activity will increase lymph flow, therefore helping to reduce swelling.

Skin care

- Keep skin clean and moisturised.
- Skin brushing should be always up the limbs towards the body. This can help keep the skin healthy and help to reduce swelling.
- Keep skin intact by avoiding cuts, scratches, insect bites, injections, acupuncture and blood samples being taken on the affected limb.
- If possible, blood pressure should not be taken on the affected limb.

General

- There are many rules and guidelines to follow for lymphoedema patients – all for valid reasons – but these can be broken occasionally as long as done carefully and infrequently so as not to compromise the progress already achieved.
- MLD can help most sufferers. In some cases, an MLD therapist would require consent to treat you from your doctor if you are currently under their care.

Contacts

MLD UK is a good source of qualified and regulated therapists
www.mlduk.org

Lymphoedema Support Network (LSN) is an excellent central source of information, support groups and general advice for suffers with many local groups actively supporting fellow sufferers:
www.lymphoedema.org

GLOSSARY

Adjuvant chemotherapy Additional cancer treatment given after primary treatment to lower the risk that the cancer will come back.

Bilateral breast cancer Breast cancer that is diagnosed in both breasts at the same time, or in the other breast within a few months of the first cancer.

Biopsy The removal, by a tiny incision through the skin and a large needle, of a small core of tissue to be examined under the microscope.

BPV (benign positional vertigo) The result of a disturbance inside the inner ear. It develops when small crystals of calcium carbonate travel from another part of the ear to the semi-circular canal, or when crystals form in the semi-circular canal itself.

Cannula A hollow, small plastic tube that is inserted into a vein to take blood or give drugs or an intravenous drip. It can stay in place for several days at a time if necessary.

Chemotherapy Drugs that are given to treat cancer but they can affect any tissue that has rapid growth, such as hair follicles, skin and the gut. It is given in the event of cancer spread, to kill the remaining cells. Even if all the obvious cancer cells have been removed, chemotherapy can reduce the likelihood of a recurrence.

Citalopram An SSRI (selective serotonin reuptake inhibitor) antidepressant.

Cone beam CT A medical imaging technique that consists of X-ray computer tomography (CT) where the X-rays are divergent, forming a cone.

Herceptin A drug that blocks the HER2 receptors found in some forms of breast cancer. It can prolong survival in patients with disease that has spread, and reduce the rate of recurrence by 50 per cent in some cases.

HER2 A protein on the surface of some cancer cells. Some breast cancers have more HER2 receptors than others. These tumours tend to grow more quickly than other types of breast cancer and respond to the drug Herceptin.

Histology The examination of tissue under the microscope, to ascertain the precise type of cell that has become malignant.

Intravenous Going directly into the blood circulation via a vein.

Lymph nodes Small glands throughout the body that cancer cells migrate to first.

Lymphoedema A condition that causes swelling in the body's tissue caused by damage to the lymphatic system from cancer treatment or problems with the lymphatic system from birth.

Mast cells A cell filled with basophil granules (a type of white cell) found in connective tissue and releasing histamine and other substances during inflammatory and allergic reactions.

Mastectomy The surgical removal of the entire breast and nipple.

Metastases Spread of the cancer from its primary site to somewhere else in the body, bones, organs, etc.

Necrosis The death of most or all the cells in an organ or tissue due to disease, injury or failure of the blood supply.

Oncologist A doctor specialising in the care of cancer patients.

Oncotype Dx This test really helps with assessing the risk of recurrence by looking at the way in which 25 genes are switched on or off in the biopsy sample. It helps in decision making as to whether chemotherapy is necessary in borderline cases. It's not for all women and it's of no value in patients with secondary cancer.

Polypharmacy The use of multiple medications at the same time.

Primary cancer Cancer that has not spread beyond the original site of the tumour/s or surrounding area.

Psychologist A person who is trained in the scientific study of people, the mind and behaviour. Psychologists can be academics and/or clinicians.

Radiologist A doctor specialising in medical imaging; that is, X-rays, ultrasound, CT and MRI scans.

Radiotherapy The use of radiation to treat cancer.

Sarcoma An uncommon cancer that can affect the body externally or internally. It can occur in, for example, muscles, bones, tendons, blood vessels and fatty tissues.

Secondary breast cancer *See* **metastases**.

Stable cancer This term is used to describe a tumour that is neither growing nor shrinking. Precisely, that it has not doubled in size or decreased by more than 30 per cent.

Tamoxifen An oestrogen receptor blocker. If the cancer cells have oestrogen receptors, this drug reduces the likelihood of a recurrence.

Zoladex An injectable drug. Peri-menopausal women with oestrogen-sensitive breast tumours can be given this in order to stop their ovaries producing oestrogen. It is also used as a hormonal therapy to treat prostate cancer.

REFERENCES

Alexis, O. and Worsley, A.J. (2018) 'A meta-synthesis of qualitative studies exploring men's sense of masculinity post-prostate cancer treatment.' *Cancer Nursing 41*, 4, 298–310.

Armenian, S.H., Xu, L., Ky, B., Sun, C., *et al.* (2016) 'Cardiovascular disease among survivors of adult-onset cancer: A community-based retrospective cohort study.' *Journal of Clinical Oncology: Official Journal of the American Society of Clinical Oncology 34*, 10, 1122–1130. Available at www.ncbi.nlm.nih.gov/pubmed/26834065

Blennerhassett, M. (2008) *Nothing Personal: Disturbing Undercurrents in Cancer Care.* Boca Raton, FL: CRC Press.

Budish, E., Roin, B.N. and Williams, H. (2015) 'Do firms underinvest in long-term research? Evidence from cancer clinical trials.' *American Economic Review 105*, 7, 2044–2085. Available at www.ncbi.nlm.nih.gov/pmc/articles/PMC4557975/

Cancer Research UK (2015) '1 in 2 people in the UK will get cancer.' Press release, 4 February. Available at www.cancerresearchuk.org/about-us/cancer-news/press-release/2015-02-04-1-in-2-people-in-the-uk-will-get-cancer

Chan, S.W., Tulloch, E., Cooper, E.S., Smith, A., *et al.* (2017) 'Montgomery and informed consent: Where are we now?' *BMJ 357*, j2224. Available at www.bmj.com/content/357/bmj.j2224

Chitnis, X., Steventon, A., Glaser, A. and Bardsley, M. (2014) *Use of Health and Social Care by People with Cancer.* Research Report. London: Nuffield Trust.

Crompton, S. (2018) 'Mind the gap! Who cares for patients once treatment is over?' *Cancerworld*, 25 May. Available at http://cancerworld.net/systems-services/mind-the-gap-who-should-help-patients-with-long-term-effects-and-how/

Daubney, M. (2015) 'Psychologists should lead the way on male mental health issues.' *The Telegraph*, 26 June. Available at www.telegraph.co.uk/men/thinking-man/11699024/Psychologists-should-lead-the-way-on-male-mental-health-issues.html

Doward, J. (2015) 'Let's reach out to men to halt shocking suicide rate.' *The Guardian*, 31 October. Available at www.theguardian.com/society/2015/oct/31/social-media-campaign-male-suicide

Galgut, C. (2006) 'Working through breast cancer.' *Therapy Today*.

Galgut, C. (2007a) 'Is it coming back? Living on a knife edge after breast cancer.' *Breast Cancer Care News*, Winter 2007/2008. Available at www.emotionalsupportthroughbreastcancer.co.uk/Is%20it%20coming%20back%20Breast%20Cancer%20Care%20News%202007.pdf

Galgut, C. (2007b) 'The psychological impact of breast cancer assessed: The testimony of a psychotherapist and breast cancer sufferer.' *Self & Society: An International Journal for Humanistic Psychology* 35, 1, 5–19.

Galgut, C. (2007c) 'Breast cancer: Therapist on the other side.' *The Times, Body and Soul*, 10 November.

Galgut C. (2008) 'Life after primary breast cancer: Changes to self and implications for relationships.' *Self & Society: An International Journal for Humanistic Psychology* 35, 6, 5–18.

Galgut, C. (2010) *The Psychological Impact of Breast Cancer: A Psychologist's Insights as a Patient.* Boca Raton, FL: CRC Press.

Galgut, C. (2011) 'On being a patient.' *Private Practice*, Winter, 8–11. Available at www.bacp.co.uk/bacp-journals/private-practice/winter-2011/

Galgut, C. (2012a) 'Trauma: Challenging the myths.' *Private Practice*, Winter, 10–14.

Galgut, C. (2012b) 'The long-term effects of treatment for breast cancer.' *Healthcare Counselling and Psychotherapy Journal* 12, 1, 31–35. Available at www.emotionalsupportthroughbreastcancer.co.uk/HCPJ%20Long%20term%20effects%20of%20treatment%20for%20breast%20cancer%202012.pdf

Galgut, C. (2013a) *Emotional Support Through Breast Cancer: A Handbook.* Boca Raton, FL: CRC Press.

Galgut, C. (2013b) 'Continuing to work after my mother's death.' *Healthcare Counselling and Psychotherapy Journal* 13, 1, 20–22. Available at www.cordeliagalgut.co.uk/Continuing_To_Work.pdf

Galgut, C. (2013c) 'Breast cancer: The emotional fallout.' *Good Housekeeping*, 7 October. Available at www.goodhousekeeping.com/uk/news/a531001/breast-cancer-the-emotional-fallout/

Galgut, C. (2013d) 'After cancer: When the effects endure.' *The Guardian*, 18 September. Available at www.theguardian.com/society/2013/sep/18/effects-treatment-endure-cancer

Galgut, C. (2014a) 'Emotional support through breast cancer.' The BMJ Opinion, 30 October. Available at https://blogs.bmj.com/bmj/2014/10/30/cordelia-calgut-emotional-support-through-breast-cancer/

Galgut, C. (2014b) 'On being a client through breast cancer.' Healthcare Counselling and Psychotherapy Journal, Summer, 17–20. Available at www.emotionalsupportthroughbreastcancer.co.uk/On%20being%20a%20client%20through%20breast%20cancer,%20Private%20Practice%202014.pdf

Galgut, C. (2016a) '4 things I didn't know about life after breast cancer.' Good Housekeeping, 9 March. Available at www.goodhousekeeping.com/uk/health/health-advice/a559936/life-after-breast-cancer/

Galgut, C. (2016b) 'Survived, but at what cost?' Private Practice, Autumn, 12–13. Available at www.cordeliagalgut.co.uk/BC248-Private-Practice-Autumn-2016_pg_12_13.pdf

Galgut, C. (2016c) 'Why are the long term effects of cancer so rarely talked about?' The BMJ Opinion, February. Available at https://blogs.bmj.com/bmj/2016/02/22/cordelia-galgut-why-are-the-long-term-effects-of-cancer-so-rarely-talked-about/

Goodhart, F. and Atkins, L. (2011) The Cancer Survivor's Companion: Practical Ways to Cope with Your Feelings After Cancer. London: Piatkus.

Gravis, G., Marino, P., Joly, F., Oudard, S., et al. (2014) 'Patients' self-assessment versus investigators' evaluation in a phase III trial in non-castrate metastatic prostate cancer (GETUG-AFU 15).' European Journal of Cancer 50, 5, 953–962. Available at www.sciencedirect.com/science/article/pii/S0959804913010307

Haines, S. (2016) Trauma Is Really Strange. London and Philadelphia, PA: Singing Dragon.

Hoffman, R.M., Lo, M., Clark, J.A., Albertsen, P.C., et al. (2017) 'Treatment decision regret among long-term survivors of localized prostate cancer: Results from the Prostate Cancer Outcomes Study.' Journal of Clinical Oncology: Official Journal of the American Society of Clinical Oncology 35, 20, 2306–2314. Available at https://ascopubs.org/doi/full/10.1200/JCO.2016.70.6317

Jang, J.W., Drumm, M.R., Efstathiou, J.A., Paly, J.J., et al. (2017) 'Long-term quality of life after definitive treatment for prostate cancer: Patient-reported outcomes in the second posttreatment decade.' Cancer Medicine 6, 7, 1827–1836. Available at https://onlinelibrary.wiley.com/doi/10.1002/cam4.1103

Kong, E.-H., Deatrick, J.A. and Bradway, C.K. (2017) 'Men's experiences after prostatectomy: A meta-synthesis.' *International Journal of Nursing Studies* 74, 161–171. Available at www.journalofnursingstudies.com/article/S0020-7489(17)30165-7/fulltext

Lloyd, C. (2018) *Grief Demystified: An Introduction.* London: Jessica Kingsley Publishers.

Macmillan Cancer Support (2013a) *Cured – But at What Cost? Long-Term Consequences of Cancer and its Treatment.* July. Available at www.macmillan.org.uk/images/cured-but-at-what-cost-report_tcm9-295213.pdf

Macmillan Cancer Support (2013b) *Throwing Light on the Consequences of Cancer and its Treatments.* July. Available at www.macmillan.org.uk/documents/aboutus/research/researchandevaluationreports/throwinglightontheconsequencesofcanceranditstreatment.pdf

Macmillan Cancer Support (2016) '1 in 5 people who return to work after cancer face discrimination.' 7 November. Available at www.macmillan.org.uk/aboutus/news/latest_news/1-in-5-people-who-return-to-work-after-cancer-face-discrimination.aspx

Macmillan Cancer Support (2017) *Am I Meant to Be Okay Now? Stories of Life After Cancer.* March–April. Available at www.macmillan.org.uk/images/LWBC-Report-2017_tcm9-317400.pdf

Macmillan Cancer Support (2019) 'Statistics fact sheet.' Updated February 2019. Available at www.macmillan.org.uk/images/cancer-statistics-factsheet_tcm9-260514.pdf

Macmillan Cancer Support and YouGov (2010) 'Facts and figures: Working through cancer.' Available at www.macmillan.org.uk/documents/aboutus/newsroom/factsheets2011/workingthroughcancerfactsheet.pdf

Sharma, S.P. (2008) 'High suicide rate among cancer patients fuels prevention discussions.' *Journal of the National Cancer Institute* 100, 24, 1750–1752. Available at https://academic.oup.com/jnci/article/100/24/1750/2607270

Watson, E., Shinkins, B., Frith, E., Neal, D., et al. (2015) 'Symptoms, unmet needs, psychological well-being and health status in survivors of prostate cancer: Implications for redesigning follow-up.' *BJU International* 117, 6b, E10–E19. Available at https://onlinelibrary.wiley.com/doi/full/10.1111/bju.13122

Wilson, B. (2018) Online Community, Macmillan Cancer Support. Available at https://community.macmillan.org.uk/

Working with Cancer (2017) 'Cancer at work: An interview with Barbara Wilson.' 28 April. Available at www.workingwithcancer.co.uk/2017/04/cancer-at-work-an-interview-with-barbara-wilson/

RESOURCES

This list is not exhaustive, and much more information is given on these websites that might be of use. Support is available below for those with both a primary and secondary diagnosis.

 While certain organisations, for example, Macmillan Cancer Support, Breast Cancer Care and several others listed below are increasingly focusing on the needs of those coping with long-term effects, others may not yet be doing so. As this book repeatedly points out, long-term effects need much more attention than they are currently getting.

Despite not all cancers being represented in the list below (listed alphabetically), Macmillan Cancer Support, for example, offers support to everyone with cancer, no matter which cancer.

Organisations

Beating Bowel Cancer, support for those affected by bowel cancer
Tel: 020 8973 0011

Bloodwise, UK specialist blood cancer charity
Tel: 0808 2080 888
https://bloodwise.org.uk

The Brain Tumour Charity, offers support to those affected
Tel: 0808 800 0004
thebraintumourcharity.org

Breast Cancer Care, provides care, information and support to people affected by breast cancer, including those living with a secondary diagnosis
Tel: 0808 800 6000
www.breastcancercare.org.uk

Breast Cancer Now, dedicated to funding research into breast cancer
https://breastcancernow.org

British Lymphology Society (BLS), provides a strong professional voice and support for those involved in the care and treatment of people with lymphoedema and related lymphatic disorders, including lipoedema
https://thebls.com

Cancer Research UK, for anyone affected by any cancer of any sort
Tel: 0808 800 4040
www.cancerresearchuk.org

Cancer.Net, provides information about the late effects of cancer
www.cancer.net

Cancer Support Community, global network offering cancer support and information
www.cancersupportcommunity.org

CLIC Sargent, UK cancer charity for children, young people and their families
Tel: 0300 330 0803
www.clicsargent.org.uk

Jo's Cervical Cancer Trust, UK charity dedicated to women, their families and friends affected by cervical cancer and cervical abnormalities
Tel: 0808 802 8000
www.jostrust.org.uk

Leukaemia Care, provides emotional support to anyone affected by a blood cancer
Tel: 0808 801 0 444
www.leukaemiacare.org.uk

Look Good Feel Better, a worldwide cancer support charity that provides practical support for women struggling with the side effects of treatment
Tel: 01372 747 500
www.lookgoodfeelbetter.co.uk

Lymphoedema Support Network (LSN), a registered charity run by people who live with lymphoedema
Tel: 020 7351 4480
www.lymphoedema.org

Macmillan Cancer Support, offers a wide variety of information and support for people living with cancer in the UK, including for those living with a secondary diagnosis. It also has an online community at community.macmillan.org.uk
Tel: 0808 808 00 00
www.macmillan.org.uk

Maggie's Centres, offer free practical, emotional and social support to people with cancer and their families and friends
Tel: 0300 123 1801
www.maggiescentres.org

Northern Ireland Cancer Network, NHS-run and includes information for people living with a terminal illness
Tel: 02890 565860
https://nican.hscni.net

Orchid – Fighting Male Cancer, exists to save men's lives from testicular, prostate and penile cancers through research and promoting awareness
https://orchid-cancer.org.uk

Pancreatic Cancer UK, offers information and support as well as research

www.pancreaticcancer.org.uk

Prostate Cancer UK, top priority is funding research to stop prostate cancer killing men

https://prostatecanceruk.org/

RipRap, information for teenagers who have a parent with cancer

www.riprap.org.uk

Roy Castle Lung Cancer Foundation, the Roy Castle lung cancer charity

www.roycastle.org

Teenage Cancer Trust, provides specialised nursing care and support for young people with cancer

Tel: 020 7612 0370

www.teenagecancertrust.org

Tenovus, provides treatment, emotional support and practical advice to those with cancer

Tel: 0808 808 1010

www.tenovuscancercare.org.uk

Counselling and psychotherapy organisations

Although the following are UK-based organisations, there are similar ones in other English-speaking countries as well as in other non-English speaking countries across the world. It is also easy to search on the internet and find therapists across the world.

British Association for Behavioural & Cognitive Psychotherapies (BABCP)

www.babcp.com

British Association for Counselling and Psychotherapy (BACP)
www.bacp.co.uk

British Psychological Society (BPS)
www.bps.org.uk

United Kingdom Council for Psychotherapy (UKCP)
www.psychotherapy.org.uk

Support available from organisations

Whether you are the person going back to work after or with cancer, a person struggling to work years after a cancer diagnosis, an employer, colleague, family member, etc., the list of organisations and their websites below might well help inform and support you, to a greater or lesser extent.

Macmillan Cancer Support helps people with a wide range of cancers and has a central landing page on their website on 'work and cancer'. This has links to large amounts of advice and guidance
www.macmillan.org.uk/about-us/what-we-do/how-we-work/work-and-cancer#262343

Barbara Wilson's website has a number of relevant articles
www.workingwithcancer.co.uk
Barbara has also written a number of pertinent blogs
https://community.macmillan.org.uk

There are other organisations whose advice is specific to particular cancers, for example, **Breast Cancer Care**
www.breastcancercare.org.uk/about-us/news-personal-stories/my-story-going-back-work

Prostate Cancer UK
https://prostatecanceruk.org/about-us/news-and-views/2014/2/going-back-to-work-with-prostate-cancer

In the UK, **Maggie's Centres** provide courses for both individuals and employers on returning to work after cancer treatment
www.maggiescentres.org/how-maggies-can-help/help-available/practical-support/returning-to-work-after-cancer

Books

Books that offer realistic or indeed any support to people coping with long-term emotional and physical effects after cancer are thin on the ground. Although I have searched everywhere I can think to search, there is little I have found that mentions 'longer-term effects' other than a few months after diagnosis or surgery, etc. There was a funny moment when I saw a book on Amazon.com that looked relevant, and then I realised it was my own forthcoming book – this one – flagged up months before publication. That's how bad the situation is! Websites for organisations such as those listed above are the best source of support I can currently find.

The book that I cited in footnote 3 in the Introduction that I consider complements this book well is called *The Cancer Survivor's Companion: Practical Ways to Cope with Your Feelings After Cancer* by Dr Frances Goodhart and Lucy Atkins. While I hope my book offers different ways of looking at the issue of long-term effects that are supportive to both those suffering them and those working with those coping longer-term, and I do include practical support, my book cannot claim to be a self-help book.

The Cancer Survivor's Companion (Goodhart and Atkins 2011) is the only self-help book focusing on cancer that I am aware of that offers in-depth, good practical support for people across a range of cancers and that also embraces the longer-term problems. As the authors say early on in their book, it is a useful resource for anyone who is living beyond diagnosis, 'whether it's days, months or years since your treatment has ended. It should be helpful whether you are feeling a little bit daunted, or completely adrift.'

My own book, *Emotional Support Through Breast Cancer: A Handbook* (CRC Press, 2013) offers breast cancer specific support.

INDEX